I WISH I WERE ENGULFED IN FLAMES

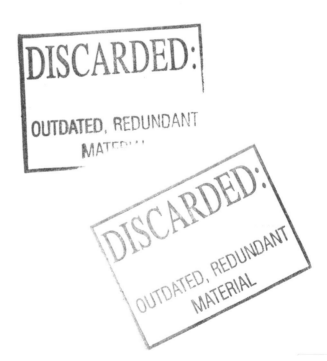

I WISH I WERE ENGULFED IN FLAMES

MY INSANE LIFE RAISING TWO BOYS WITH AUTISM

JENI DECKER

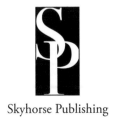

Skyhorse Publishing

Skyhorse Publishing books may be purchased in bulk at special discounts for sales promotion, corporate gifts, fund-raising, or educational purposes. Special editions can also be created to specifications. For details, contact the Special Sales Department, Skyhorse Publishing, 307 West 36th Street, 11th Floor, New York, NY 10018 or info@skyhorsepublishing.com.

Skyhorse® and Skyhorse Publishing® are registered trademarks of Skyhorse Publishing, Inc.®, a Delaware corporation.

Visit our website at www.skyhorsepublishing.com.

10 9 8 7 6 5 4 3 2 1

Library of Congress Cataloging-in-Publication Data available on file.
ISBN: 978-1-61608-485-1

Printed in the United States of America

*If a man does not keep pace with his companions,
perhaps it is because he hears a different drummer.
Let him step to the music he hears,
however measured or far away.*

—Henry David Thoreau, 1854

Contents

Tickling the Weiner

"Stars."

"Stars?"

"Stars, yes." When Jaxson smiles, he lights up a room. Other times, he resembles the devil incarnate.

"Stars?"

It went back and forth like that for two minutes. He wanted something from me and if I couldn't figure out what he wanted in the next twenty seconds or so, shit would be hitting the fan—or the walls. Biting, hitting, screaming, kicking—any or all of the above were imminent.

He was doing his part—he was asking. I just wasn't equal to the task. I had no idea what stars meant in his strange little world. He could literally want something having to do with a star, or the word he was saying could *sound* like star, or he could just as easily mean pumpernickel bread.

"Stars . . . " I could see it bubbling up within him, that sense of urgency. I felt for the little guy. He tilted his head, thinking a minute, the synapses firing in his special brain.

"DS?" he inquired.

DS? DS? Wait . . .

DS! Eureka! Nintendo DS. He wanted his game!

"DS? You want your DS?"

What stars had to do with the DS I had no idea.

"DS, please."

You have to love a little autistic kid prone to fits who can still use the word please. Mind you, he doesn't understand anything about social graces—he's just parroting the word because I've said it a million times when he asks for something. But, if he's going to vibrate through life snatching food from people's plates like Helen Keller before meeting Annie Sullivan, he's at least going to say please when he does it.

I grabbed his face, covering it with kisses as he pulled away. He was happy I finally understood him, but not as pleased with the sudden facial attention. That's another issue, being touched. He doesn't like it much. I do it anyway. My reasoning is that he'll somehow get desensitized by it—or not. Either way, I'd earned the right. After nine months of morning sickness and an all-night labor session, you get to kiss the kid as much as you want. At least when they're still lacking pubic and armpit hair. Once they become hirsute beings, all bets are off.

The next problem was that Jake, Jaxson's older brother, had the DS. Earlier, Jake had thrown his own DS against the wall and it broke, so he'd taken to his room with the only other one in the house. Yes, I know. I can hear the judgmental sighs and see the eyes rolling now. Don't criticize me till you've lived in my private Idaho, where things are likely to come flying across the room at any moment, whacking you in the temple.

Jake is my first son, who also has autism. Jake also can't tell a lie. Whenever he does something bad, he tells me about it immediately. For this reason, I think all people should have a touch of autism. Truth in advertising—you know what you're getting.

I knocked on Jake's locked door and heard some shuffling and odd little sounds coming from within. As long as the room's not on fire and the floor isn't littered with bomb-making materials, that's all I need to know.

I do know, however, that as of late, he's prone to "tickling his wiener." I know this because he tells me every time he does it, much to my motherly chagrin.

Earlier that day at school they showed Jake's fifth grade class one of those health movies where they separate the boys and girls and each group views a movie about their developing bodies. The girls get to discuss their periods, and the boys get to talk about impending hair growth and masturbation. I wasn't that worried about the "lesson." I was expecting the old "boys have a penis, girls have a vagina" routine, and I'd already taught Jake that when he was five. I knew it had sunk in because at that plucky age, he'd announced it to the entire deli department at our Wal-Mart Super Center. Two other moms in line behind me had been amused, though the senior citizen couple in front of me looked considerably less . . . charmed. The wife, obviously an old church lady, had turned around and I'd seen it in her eyes: I was the white trash vixen wearing blue eyeliner and my kids were a weekend away from being permanent wards of the state.

But apparently we've come a long way since I saw the fifth grade movie because when Jake eventually opened his bedroom door, he said, "Mom, the man said everyone does it . . . the wiener tickle thing."

"He did?" What man? The gym teacher? That weird-looking science teacher with the comb over, or some other smarmy *vicieuse*? Is there a pedophiliac teacher on staff that I'm as yet unaware of?

"The doctor who gave the speech."

Phew. A doctor. Sure, he's a man, but he's got a medical degree. He's been sanctioned to discuss the penis with young men.

"So, what did he call it?"

"Penis."

"Ah."

"Did the boys laugh?"

Jake grinned. "Some."

"Did you?"

He was doing that thing where he smiled nervously but then tried to keep from smiling. "No, but I wanted to." Jake tore his face from the floor and looked right at me, something he didn't often do. He and eye contact are not best mates.

"He said everybody does it sometimes. In private."

Duly noted. It's officially okay to tickle your wiener as long as you do it in private.

Then it happened. I could see it on his face—the act of putting two and two together as kids eventually do, to our parental horror— matching a fact to a possibility and sliding deftly into home plate.

"Do you?"

"Huh?" Surely the phone was ringing somewhere in the house.

"Do you do it? Tickle your . . . " His voice trailed off as he broke eye contact and squeezed his eyes shut, clearly torn between wanting to know the answer and imagining his mother with a vagina.

Isn't that a pot boiling over on the stove? Or possibly an impending natural disaster of some kind? Perhaps there's a band of Jehovah's Witnesses on the front porch waiting to give testimony.

"... oh, you don't have one." He was rounding third and I could feel a case of anxiety hives in my not-so-distant future.

I scratched the back of my neck, hoping the line of questioning would end.

"Do you tickle your vagina?"

Oh, Christ on a cracker, where's that frigging tornado when you need it? I'd welcome the roof flying off of the house right about now. I have insurance, and frankly, every closet in my home is well past the point of saving with a spring cleaning. If the entire contents of my home were suddenly sucked into the sky and spread around the fifty acres we lived on, I could start afresh.

New house, new closets, new clutter.

"Well, I ... uh ... "

Jake's got a pretty well-honed BS detector. I can't fake it, like an orgasm. Either I tell him the truth—and that's not gonna happen—or I need a distraction pretty darned quick, because here's the thing:

I'd sooner stick a finger up my nose, pull out a glob of snot and wipe it all over David Sedaris' face during a book signing in the middle of a Barnes and Noble than admit to *that* aloud.

It's just not done.

But saving grace was on his way, in the form of Jaxson running through the living room screaming like a banshee, plastic golf club in one hand over his head and a look of ominous displeasure on his crumpled face.

"DS!"

Jake instantly forgot about my vagina and ran for the safety of his bedroom. He slammed the door and left me to deal with the flailing golf pro in full tantrum mode.

I believe that was the first and only time in my life I welcomed an autistic meltdown—while taking the business end of a plastic golf putter to the head.

"Jake! Bring me the DS!" I screamed.

It's a perfect snapshot of my life.

Bob and weave, baby. Bob and weave.

Can Someone Choke Themselves with Their Bare Hands?

I straddle my son, holding his wrists down, hoping he'll calm down enough so that I can get off him. I need an ibuprofen. He's in the middle of one of his tantrums and he's all over the place—one moment kicking me in the stomach, the next moment, patting me on the head.

"You okay, Mom? S'okay."

I love you, I hate you, I love you, I hate you. I then take a head-butt to the nose and it's lights out for a few seconds. Tiny white specs flood my field of vision and I crumple to the floor with Jaxson still clinging to me. I start sobbing and don't stop for a good half hour.

I stare at my reflection in the shards of broken Christmas bulbs next to me—the blank look I see refracted back is disturbing. I've disappeared into myself like a snail pulling back into its protective shell.

So that's what post-traumatic stress looks like.

This is me, Jeni: I'm five-foot nuthin', one hundred and . . . *ahem* pounds—a roly-poly, forty-something, Rubenesque bon-bon of a gal, often described as cute but never sexy. I have two autistic children, an Australian shepherd named Sugar, and an albino frog named Humbert Humbert.

I've also got a husband, but he's sort of a bit player in the melodrama that is my life. The frog gets more screen time than he does, mostly because the frog is physically present in the house more than my husband. The frog can't escape. The husband can.

We moved from Florida to Michigan in 2007 (from a small neighborhood to a fifty-acre farm) because my mother had recently bought property and offered to help us build a home. She knew I needed help—I had a nine-year-old with severe OCD and major socialization issues, a five-year-old who was barely verbal, physically aggressive, and not anywhere near being toilet trained, and a husband who was having a difficult time dealing with his two disabled children.

The only tool I had at my disposal was a prescription for an anti-depressant.

What I had, essentially, was a mess.

Now it's Christmas Eve, 2008—the year was coming to an end, not unlike my sanity.

My husband had gone out for a bit of last minute holiday shopping, leaving me with twelve-year-old Jake to obsessively pummel me with random questions, while eight-year-old Jaxson did the same with his fists.

I was praying Santa would drop by early to deliver some sort of legal pharmaceutical magic I could sprinkle over Jaxson to knock him out for an hour—or five.

He ran around the room yanking pictures off the walls, knocking over tables and chairs, screaming at the top of his lungs, and clawing at me whenever I came near him.

Christmas break sucks. Take my kids off their schedules, even if part of that schedule includes school—which they both hate—and things begin to deteriorate fairly quickly.

Jaxson wanted to go outside and play in the snow. I was preparing for Mom and Bob to arrive for dinner and trying to clean the house. During the four hours that my husband disappeared to "shop," I had to employ the kind of physical prowess only high school wrestlers are familiar with.

After he tossed a picture from the wall at me, I lunged at Jaxson, straddling his waist. I held both of his wrists to the carpet and waited out his flailing and kicking until he became tired enough that I could safely get off him. Then he cried and took to my bedroom, hiding under the covers on my bed. I left him in my room but brought a heavy dose of guilt with me as I hurried to clean the toilets and make a salad.

After I washed my hands, of course.

Jake, the Official Hygiene Ambassador, was keeping an eye on me in that regard, all while following me around the house, tossing questions at me like live grenades.

"I just need some proof, Mom. I need some straight answers. So I'm gonna leave cookies out for Santa, and if he's not real, the cookies won't be eaten, right?" We'd already had *the talk* but Jake was still grasping at the magical thinking we're all guilty of when we don't like the answer reality provides.

"Okay, then. Hand me that spray bleach."

He passed me the cleaner. "You won't eat them, right?"

I wiped the hair from my eyes with the side of my forearm, making sure to keep my chemically dirty hands away from my face. "What are you looking for here, honey? The truth, or something that will make you feel better?"

Jake eyed me suspiciously, and then headed for his room. "Never mind. I don't want to talk about it. Just don't eat the cookies."

I got a five minute respite wherein all I had to deal with was the cleanliness of the toilet. Then Jaxson had re-entered the scene, threw himself on the floor beneath me, and began to scream as I cleaned the bathroom. I ignored him, scrub, scrub, scrubbing Christmas Eve into oblivion.

Jingle Bells, Jingle Bells . . . I hummed with alarming ferocity, hoping it would drown out the little guy wailing at the top of his lungs.

It was not long before Jake returned with more questions, yelling over his still screaming brother.

"Can someone choke themselves with their bare hands?" Jake had both hands wrapped tightly around his throat, his face becoming redder by the second.

"I don't know. Give it a go and let me know how it turns out."

Scrub, scrub, flush. Clean toilet: Check.

Jake trusts no one. The entire world and its contents are conspiring to make his life miserable or cause him physical harm.

"What about a fork? Is it possible to swallow a fork?" Jake yelled over his brother, who was now pounding the nearby wall with his little feet.

"I'm pretty sure you can't swallow a fork," I screamed, stepping over Jaxson. I headed for the other bathroom with Jake following me.

It took Jaxson a minute to realize he wasn't center stage. Once he did, he got up, found us in the other bathroom, and threw himself another tot-sized tantrum.

"I so mad!" Jaxson announced, climbing into the empty bathtub.

"If I create my virtual world, jump into the TV and start playing with Mario, what happens if the electricity goes out? Will I be stuck in the virtual world, forever?" Jake leaned his head against the door frame as I bent over my second commode of the day, trying not to pass out from the noxious chemical fumes.

Jake's newest brainchild was some sort of virtual world he thought he could persuade the scientific community to invent. He'd recently made me send out a mass email with the following:

Dear Computer Geniuses and Scientists,

I want a world called the virtual world. You put on a helmet and I want it to be the realest graphics you can make. It can link to any game system and when it accidentally turns off, you can still take off the helmet. And make a screen so people outside the virtual world can watch you.

Sincerely, Jake
PS—Make it very realistic

Of course, this email never got sent. I'd typed the letter, added the entire contents of my address book to the *Send To* column as Jake hovered over my shoulder, and then pretended to click send when he went to the kitchen for a soda.

Jake stared at me as I scoured the toilet bowl, patiently awaiting a response.

"I can only say that if you invent this virtual world, that's something you might need to look into."

Lately Jake had been obsessing more and more. I began to wonder if a trip to the pediatrician to check into some sort of medication might be in order. He couldn't even go a few minutes without bombarding me with a plethora of questions, one right after the other, faster than I was able to answer. It was starting to interfere with his daily life.

Not to mention mine.

It was like I imagined a stun gun attack would feel: *Zap!*— a moment of disorientation followed by a slow recovery. Only in this scenario, I'd be zapped again as soon as my eyes stopped rolling back in my head.

"Mom, I hate school. I wish they would just send me to juvie."

Bang, bang, bang! Jaxson kicked the side of the tub, tossing shampoo bottles overboard.

"No you don't. People would touch all your stuff, you wouldn't have wipies to clean your butt with, and you'd have to sleep alone. You wouldn't do well in juvie, Jake."

Yank! Down went the basket of towels. When Jax saw my expression, he flew out of the tub and exited the bathroom, leaving a trail of knocked-over items in his wake.

"Mom?" Jake began, tentatively.

"What, honey?" I continued to ignore Jaxson, trying to give Jake my full attention—well, him *and* the area behind the toilet bowl that rarely got any attention of its own.

"Fear is an emotion God shouldn't have given us. Because we still have common sense."

I didn't realize the profundity of this statement until I'd thought about it for a minute. "That's very smart, Jake."

"Maybe I could build a machine that would take away fear. After I get my virtual world helmet made."

Crash! Something that sounded suspiciously like glass fell in the other room.

"Uh, huh . . . " You get right on that. "Interesting idea, honey."

Realizing the bathroom was as clean as it was going to get, I headed off to find out what was broken in the other room, hoping Jax didn't need stitches.

"Mom, who is more irritating, me or Jaxson?"

I stood over a broken Christmas bulb on the kitchen floor. "You both have your moments."

"What do I do that's as bad as his fits?"

Jake held the dustpan for me and I swept up the mess as Jaxson watched from across the room. I looked up at him, pointed my finger and said, "Bad boy," before jumping back into the interrogation with my elder son.

"You ask lots of questions. Questions, questions, questions. Questions are good, but sometimes when they're coming as fast and furious as you ask them—"

"No bad boy. No!" Jaxson screamed, and again ran to hide under the covers on my bed.

"—it feels just like getting hit with one of your brother's little fists. Or a stun gun." I took a deep breath and exhaled, trying not to cry.

"I guess God just made me more curious than normal people. I'm bi-curious."

I smiled. "Where did you hear that word?"

"On TV somewhere," Jake picked up a few stray shards of red glass.

At last, finally I got everything done that needed to be done and was finally able to sit in the rocking chair with Jaxson and make nice. Usually, when he realizes he isn't going to get his way, there is a hurricane of dysfunctional behavior followed by a self-imposed time out, then him hugging me and crying, eventually leading to, "Better, Ruby?"

He calls me Ruby and I call him Max, something that started when I began mimicking the voice of the cartoon character on *Max & Ruby,* one of his favorite shows.

"Yes, Max. All better," I squeaked in my cartoon voice.

"Good job, Ruby." Jaxson smiled and used his little fingers to push the downturned corners of my mouth up into a smile.

I wanted to scream, was seconds away from sobbing violently, but I'd just told him it was all better so I needed him to see on my face that it was.

Autistic people often have a problem matching a facial expression with a corresponding emotion. All through elementary school, Jake regularly had to consult the Chart of Expressions on his special needs classroom wall in order to know what someone he was talking to might be feeling inside.

On this Christmas Eve, if my emotional state had been portrayed on the Chart of Expressions, it would have included two slits for eyes, a large O for a mouth, and a dialogue bubble that said: "Somebody kill me before this gets any worse!"

When their father finally returned home, Jaxson was gearing up for another fit.

I heard my husband mumble under his breath, "I can't wait until this is all over."

This was him presumably referring to Christmas and all of the extra time and effort the holiday preparations necessitated. Unfortunately, Jake heard every word.

Are you kidding me?

I'll admit there were a few dangerous seconds when, if my actions had reflected my internal emotions, I'd now be incarcerated for first-degree murder and my children would be permanent wards of the state. It was during those few dangerous seconds that I fully grasped what the word *snap* means with regard to what people do in a blinding instant of rage.

The better parent in me waited until Jake had called his father *rude* and wandered off to his bedroom.

Then, I responded. Quietly, and not without a hint of vitriol. "Let me tell you something, Mister. Until you've taken two kicks to the kidney and an almost debilitating head-butt to the nose, accompanied by enough close-fisted punches to cause the ugly bruise that's certain to be on my shoulder tomorrow, I'm going to need you to *shut your mouth!*" I kept my hissing to a volume only he could hear. "While you were battling last minute shoppers, I cleaned two bathrooms, vacuumed four rooms, cleaned one kitchen, made a salad and *still* managed to deal with the little prizefighter over there, who is now dry humping his Christmas stocking!"

My husband was having "issues" coming to terms with his children's autism. Recently he'd said to me, "Well, I'd take them out, but they don't like doing anything."

My response wasn't exactly full of Christmas cheer. "Correction. They don't like doing anything *you* like. How about doing something *they* like? Jax loves playing on the swings. Jake wants to make things in the shed. You will never turn them into the little men you dreamed they'd be, so how about realizing they're perfect little men just as they are? I'm not sure who it was that told you hanging out with kids is always fun. Because I don't particularly like telling Jake his Mad Guy/Sad Guy story every night, or repeatedly casting the fishing rod for Jax so he can hold the end while I reel it in. Do you think I like spending hours of my life doing these repetitive, painfully boring things? No. But I do them because they like it. I do it for them, not for me. If you think for one minute I wouldn't prefer getting a pedicure or spending a little time alone at the library, you're mistaken, buddy. I'd settle for a nap. I don't think I've taken one in twelve years."

I could almost hear the Christmas version of my angst set to musical accompaniment as my chagrined husband sulked off to take a shower.

> *Six veggies cut up . . .*
> *Five tan-trums quelled . . .*
> *Four Xanax downed . . .*
> *Three bedrooms cleaned . . .*
> *Two bleached-out johns . . .*
> *And a spark-ling kitch-en sink!*

On some days I wonder just how harshly I'd be judged if I disappeared suddenly, changed my name, and never returned. Obviously I know the answer to this question. There would be judgment and it would be deserved. You don't just cut and run on your kids—not unless you're a complete and utter douche bag. Couple that with the fact that even though I'm not a practicing Catholic, the nuns at St. Charles Catholic School did enough damage to tattoo the religious taint of guilt on my soul forever.

Christmas Eve went fairly smoothly after that. Mom and Bob arrived for dinner, presents were revealed, the questions stopped, and there were no more tantrums.

Just before bedtime—when he'd close his eyes, lay his head on the bed next to his brother and dream of sugarplums and all that jazz—Jake entered the living room to find me staring at the television in an almost vegetative state, watching *The Nightmare Before Christmas*.

He offered an epiphany: "I think I need to forget about the swallowing the fork thing, Mom. If I don't quit thinking about it, I'll never make it in this life."

Damn, that kid is smart.

"Night, Jake."

"Night, Mom."

Merry Christmas.

Conversations with Jake

I wish I could take a poop in peace.

I was sitting in the bathroom, perusing a magazine, and trying to evacuate my bowels when Jake ran into the room with not a hint of concern for my personal space.

"I put this in my mouth."

He held out a glob of something. It was pink and gooey—something they made at school called *flubber* or *flabber* or *floozy-whatzit*.

What the hell are they up to at school these days, and why must they send this crap home for me to deal with?

I was sure there was a teaching moment in there somewhere, but was at a loss for what the lesson with the gooey substance actually entailed.

"Don't put bad things in your mouth," immediately sprang from my own, and as he walked away, I pondered the implications of my statement.

Not very specific, was I?

Bad things could be translated within Jake's mind as any number of things, and I wondered if my flippant one-liners would eventually lead to pricey therapy. What if he associated "bad things" with the private parts of another and was never able to perform certain *activities* with someone. Male or female. Because the jury was still out on that one.

Jake had done, said, and asked certain things, leading me to believe his sexuality was still up in the air.

From ages three to six, he had a collection of dolls which left me amused and his father decidedly not as tickled.

At the toy section of our local store one day, as he was about to choose his fifth doll, I asked him, "Honey, why do you want another doll? You can have any toy you want."

He looked up at me, his small face illuminated in the glow of the spinning light attached to the endcap, highlighting the most recent blue-light special. "Because they look so lonely, Mommy. They want me to take them home."

I wiped the lone tear that sprang from the corner of my eye, grabbed three dolls, shoved them into his arms, and thanked Almighty Jesus we weren't at the local animal shelter.

Then there'd been the "hairless conversation," or what I now refer to as the "Unbearable Stupidity of a Mother Distracted by Road Construction and a Hooters Billboard" incident.

I was returning home from picking up Jake and his cousin Max from elementary school, with Jaxson safely strapped into his car seat, when the older boys started play-slapping one another over the seats. Jake was in the passenger seat, Max in the rear, and they were dangerously close to spilling French fries all over the floor.

"I'm a man!" roared Max, giggling.

"No, I'm *the* man!" Jake retaliated, sending a nugget into the air and, thankfully, onto his brother's lap. Jaxson just smiled and shoved it into his mouth, as if McNuggets normally rained down from the heavens in his special world.

"That's enough," I swatted, maneuvering around a road construction crew and melding into the single line of moving traffic. "Neither of you are men. At least until you grow armpit hair."

A few minutes of silence ensued as the boys foraged in their armpits for hair.

"Mom, who else doesn't have armpit hair?" Jake asked, as he is wont to do whenever he needs to compare one situation with another to get a visual representation of "like" things. For whatever reason, that helps him cope. But, because of the giant Hooters sign looming over me and the bulbous breasts straining out of the t-shirt of the woman on the advertisement, I offered a flippant answer.

Flippancy is eventually going to get the better of me.

"Uh . . . body builders. They shave their bodies and apply oil when they perform in contests. It enhances the definition of their muscles."

I took a long sip of my iced tea as Jake pondered the validity of my answer.

"Who else?" he asked, popping a fry into his mouth.

"Swimmers!" Max offered from the back seat, smiling broadly.

"Exactly. They shave their bodies sometimes so that they can move through the water more quickly. That's why they wear those plastic caps on their heads, too."

"That makes them hydrodynamic!" Max ventured into the fray again, happy to enlighten us with a word that I wasn't even sure existed. On the off-chance that the six-year-old was more knowledgeable than I in that regard, I let it go. It wouldn't be the first time.

"Who else?" Jake could go on pondering the hairless possibilities like that forever if you let him.

And then I said it, because I was tired and wanted to get home and move the laundry from the washer to the dryer before Oprah came on.

"Drag queens."

Jake's little brow furrowed and he cocked his head, swallowing his food. "What's a drag queen?"

Jesus, Mary and Joseph.

"Yeah, what's a drag queen?" Max handed Jaxson the rest of his uneaten fries and leaned forward, his head popping out between the front seats.

I know it's a horrible thing to wonder, but at that moment, I'd have given my left butt cheek for three quiet, non-speaking children in the car, rather than just one who appeared, by the way, to have bathed in ketchup.

I sucked in a breath. "A drag queen is a man that dresses like a woman and sings songs on a stage."

That was about right, wasn't it? Not all-inclusive or entirely PC, but a nice summation, none the less.

"And shaves his armpits?" Jake asked, flummoxed.

"That is correct, sir." I used my finger to lift the lid from my drink, scooping out a few pieces of ice to chew on.

"But why would he want to do that?"

"Yeah, why Aunt Jeni?"

A piece of ice fell from my mouth to my lap as I answered, "Because hairy armpits don't go well with dresses."

"*Eeeewww*, Mom! That has your spit on it. Throw it away!" And that's all it took to distract them from the hairless armpit discussion. A germ-ridden ice cube.

I tossed the offending cube out the opened window and held my hand out for the antibacterial hand sanitizer that Jake pulled from the center console with swift urgency.

He squirted a dollop into my palm, a look of disgust on his face, the drag queen discussion now a distant memory.

Distant like the time years before when he was five and asked me, "Mom, can a man and a man get married?"

I'd been cleaning up the back porch while he played on his swing set and I stopped sweeping, resting my chin on the end of the broom handle.

"Well, yes they can," I answered because I knew he wasn't asking if two men could go down to the county courthouse and obtain a marriage license or civil ceremony certificate, or move to Canada and marry without the Jesus freaks stoning them on the way in. He wanted to know if two men could live together, love together, and have a family. So I believe I gave the appropriate response.

"Is that weird?" he asked, sitting in the swing, using a toe to dig in the dirt.

"No, nothing's weird if you don't think it is, honey."

"But is it normal?"

"What's normal?" I asked, wondering how he defined the word.

"Mom! You know what normal means!" Jake only likes to deal in facts. Black or white, right or wrong, his mind leaves no room for the possibility of fluidity in any circumstance. Yes or no answers should be given whenever possible as far as he is concerned, and the world would be a much easier place to navigate if everyone conformed to that notion.

I can't remember now how I'd defined normal that day. With Jake, there were always these discussions that left me feeling anxious and slightly nauseous. Not because of the content, but because I was always afraid I might say something that would come back to bite me or him in the ass later in life. I wanted him to make his own choices— about sexuality, about politics, about religion, about people in general. So what I tried to do was give him the most honest, age-appropriate answers I could come up with at any given moment and hope Social Services didn't come knocking on my door one afternoon. I think that's the best any parent can do.

But his most recent questioning on the topic, at age twelve, now led me to believe that I couldn't win for losing.

"Mom, can I read your book when it gets published?"

We were en route to school, and damn if I already had to deal with a hot topic.

"No, honey. It's for adults."

"What's it about?"

"It's about a young boy who leaves home when he's seventeen and lives in New York for twenty years before he returns home." The book in question was *Far From Happy*, a novel I'd recently signed a contract for. My first published work.

The protagonist was a male hustler.

"Is it like your Macy movie? With the boys kissing?"

Yes, in fact. *Macy's Wait* was a short film my mother and I had recently completed, and apparently he'd seen me editing the video, though this was the first time he'd mentioned it.

"Well, sort of. The boy is gay. Remember when I told you what gay meant?"

"Yeah, that's gross, Mom."

I had exactly nine minutes before I dropped him off in front of his middle school and I used every second of it explaining the facets of the word *tolerance* and how I didn't actually like the word, because it presumed that there was something that needed to be tolerated about another individual and I preferred to believe that we are all equal and beautiful because of our differences and no matter who someone is or what they believe, love was never wrong and it was nobody's place to judge someone else for who they loved.

As we pulled into the parking lot, I finished with this: "Now, you understand that some men love men, and some men love women, and some women love men, and some women love women, right? And any of those combinations is perfectly acceptable. It's okay that you would rather kiss a girl, but—"

"—eeeew, Mom! That's even *more* gross!" When the car door slammed and I pulled around the circle, I was shaking my head. It seemed, at that moment, kissing anyone was gross.

And that was just fine with me.

I Hate Mornings
by Jake Lopez

I hate mornings
I don't like the bus. It is noisy.
It makes me stressed in the mornings.
I don't like the way paper sounds.
It gives me the chills.
I don't like to read first thing in the morning.
I don't like the feeling of glue in the morning.
Being sticky in the mornings makes me uncomfortable.
I don't like mini-lessons because they're too short and that bothers
me.
I don't like when people rub their hands together.
It also gives me chills.
All of those things make my day bad.
I get confused when there are too many things happening.
I get very angry when I get confused.
I feel like people don't understand me sometimes.
I don't like school in the mornings.
I don't like to do so many things at once.

If Life's a Highway, I Want Off at the Next Exit

November 10, 2009
Journal note from Jake's teacher

Jake realized he has a tiny blackhead on his nose. It caused great pain for him during language arts, to the point of distraction.
Ms. D

Later that evening, Jake came out of the bathroom sniffing his hand, a disturbed look on his face. "I don't usually poop at this time of day."

Irregularity with regard to bowel movements is a concern for Jake because it's something he can't control.

"It might have something to do with those three pieces of fried chicken you just ate for dinner," I said. "Grease makes food slide right through you. And I'm pretty sure it's not helping your complexion." I wiped the grease off my own fingers and onto my sweatpants—at this point, there's not anyone even remotely concerned about me getting acne or thighs dappled with cellulite but he's got his whole life ahead of him.

"What's a complexion?" Jake asked, worried.

"Your skin. Like on your face."

"What do I do about the dot on my nose? It concerns me."

"I heard it caused you great distress in language arts class today. How did you even know it was there?"

"I was in the bathroom and I noticed it in the mirror. I couldn't concentrate the rest of the day. The dot is disturbing."

What must it feel like for him—all of these banal things festering in his mind. He can't stand the way paper feels—at school this just has to be nerve-racking. Book pages turning, papers being passed out, notes shuffling—the sensory minefield he has to wade through daily is something most people can't remotely relate to.

Picture this:

You're locked in a speeding car at night, racing down the highway at breakneck speed. It's the middle of summer—you're hot, uncomfortable and sweaty. There are sirens wailing outside and there's a baby with a stinky diaper next to you, screaming. The interior car lights flash on and off, blinding you. The radio is turned up full blast to heavy metal music. Nobody is driving—you have no control.

Now you *might* have an idea of what it's like to be autistic on any given day.

You are expected to deal with this *and* get through your normal daily routine without exploding. Add socialization issues to this and you've got a recipe for a ten car pileup on your little highway to hell.

Take, for instance, gym class. Normally, this is a place where kids can let off steam and get some exercise. But for the "sensory challenged" it's a noise salad. Sneakers squeaking against the shiny, wooden floor. Jocular roughhousing. Kids racing around one another, laughing and screaming— all under the guise of fun. Team sports only illustrate how truly unequal the autistic child actually is. Being slightly clumsy and uncomfortable in his own skin, gym only serves to exacerbate his sense of singularity.

I'm not sure who designed the game of dodgeball for example, but I am certain, the idiot wasn't autistic. Sure, let's put some poor sap in the middle of a circle and lob a ball at them while talking smack.

Smack-talk only makes Jake want to do some inappropriate smacking of his own. He doesn't get the fun in joking around while trying to dodge a ball that's headed straight for him.

In elementary school, the counselors tried to solve his sensory overload by giving him a huge set of noise-reducing headphones. Yeah, that was nice. Now he not only didn't fit in, but he had a monstrous set of yellow earphones to even further separate him from his peers. He looked like a big, sweaty bumblebee.

He might as well have had a sign on his back that said: "Kick me, please."

The yellow headphones were eventually replaced with orange ear plugs that he now wears in the gym, in the noisy hallways, and often in class. Add a mini bottle of antibacterial gel to his arsenal of protection, and all he needs is a pocket protector and a lisp and he's right out of central casting for Nerds III.

I am the Walrus, goo goo ga joob.

With Jaxson, it's different. He's blissfully unaware of even the concept of social ineptitude. He's on a stage of his own and we're all bit players, coming in now and again to offer clothing or food. At nine, he's just beginning to speak in complete sentences and still wears a diaper. The only world he knows exists within the confines of our house, his classroom, and the occasional trip to the pediatrician. His inability to communicate with others in a meaningful way makes forming relationships difficult. He's unaffected by social mores or his lack of appropriate actions because they do not exist within the production in which he's starring.

They don't exist for him *yet* anyway.

I wish they never will.

When you don't know something exists, you can't feel self-conscious about it. You can't be made to feel less than. His older brother, however, isn't so lucky.

Last night before bed, Jake asked me this:

"Mom, in Heaven will I be normal?"

Ugh. How do I answer this? And what is the truth? Mommy's truth isn't something he's apt to enjoy, because Mommy often wonders if here, where we are now, is as good as it ever gets. More and more, Mommy thinks of life as a highway and the only way to get off is running out of gas or slamming into a cement piling.

The big sleep. Click, the lights are off. Elvis has left the building.

But bedtime is definitely not the time for pessimism.

So what do I answer? "Honey, heaven is whatever each person wants it to be."

"Really?" he asks, rubbing his tired eyes.

"Yep, I'm pretty sure."

"I love you, Mom."

"I love you too, buddy. Now go to sleep."

Click. Lights out.

At Some Point, I'm Gonna Need Some Therapy

"That's not fair!" Jake whined as I shoved groceries into the opened cabinets, trying to get them in as fast as Jaxson was grabbing them and absconding to God knows where.

Chips disappeared, an entire bag of grapes— someone would be on the toilet all night.

"Fair? Really? You want to go down that road, do you? Because that's a can of worms I don't think you want to open." I was mixing my metaphors here and I was pretty sure—

"—worms? What worms?"

And we're off.

"No worms, Jake, I'm just saying that we don't want to start comparing notes on what's fair and what's—"

"—you bought a can of worms?" Jake feverishly looked around the kitchen and amid the bags of groceries. The very idea of worms in the same general proximity as the food he'd be required to eat was threatening to consume him in an oncoming tidal wave of horror.

"NO WORMS. It's a figure of speech. Forget I said it."

"So you didn't get any worms?" Clearly he didn't believe me because he was using his toe to pull the plastic bags open, trying to see into them without touching anything with his hands.

"No Jake. I did not purchase any worms. They weren't on sale today and I left my worm coupons at home."

"Then why did you say it? Why do you do that? Now I don't believe you!" He continued his search through the bags, grabbing a pair of cooking tongs and dragging bags to the center of the kitchen floor.

I sighed heavily and slammed a cabinet shut. "I don't believe myself sometimes, Jake. Truly. I have to walk on eggshells every time I open my mouth around you for Christ's sake. I'm a writer, what do you expect?"

Jake turned his attention to the floor beneath my feet. "What eggshells?"

Oh, Mary H. Magdalene!

"Never mind! Out of the kitchen. Let me finish this, will you?"

"Mom, you're weird. Really, I think you were born on another planet. You never make sense."

Suddenly I imagined myself sitting across from a smartly dressed therapist I could never afford, given the current state of the health care system in the United States.

"What do you do when you're feeling overwhelmed?" she'd ask, tapping her bottom lip with the end of her pen.

"I eat," I'd offer, brushing the errant cheese doodle crumbs from my jeans.

"That's not good for you, healthwise." She'd jot a note or two in my folder, shaking her head.

"Yeah, I'm not really looking for length of life, doc, so much as a slow, steady decline, whereby I don't even notice till I'm actually dead. I just suddenly am. I mean, I'm not seeing, generally speaking, any need to prolong the agony."

That night, Jake had lots of questions. Not his "normal" questions, but questions brought about by the worm fiasco earlier in the day.

From the moment he was born, he was never a good sleeper and I had to lie in the bed, *my bed* (yes, he still sleeps with me, what about it?), and wait for him to fall asleep before disengaging whatever body part of mine was underneath him, and perform a series of stealth movements until I extricated myself from the room to sweet, sweet freedom.

Now he has questions. Every night, before he can even try to close his eyes, he comes out of the room and asks me the same five questions. Here are my responses:

There are no legendary creatures.

The door is double locked.

There is a heaven and you're going there someday.

Yes, I'm sure.

Yes, I'll leave the light on in both bathrooms.

For the first, let's say, sixteen months of this tiptoe around hell, I prided myself on my patience as he asked each question and I gave the corresponding response. I'm not proud of this, but my patience has since waned. Now, when I hear his feet coming across the room, before he can even ask question one, this is what he hears coming from my lips in one quick succession of words that become increasingly irritated and high-pitched:

"There are no legendary creatures, the door is double locked, there is a heaven and you're going there someday, yes, I'll leave the light on in both bathrooms."

"I love you, Mom," he always replies.

"I love you too, buddy. Now go to sleep."

But tonight, we were expanding our usual repertoire, apparently.

After what he thought was a dangerous ride in the RTV out to the fields, he'd taken to his room for the remainder of the day. He'd insisted we were driving too fast— that we were in danger of careening into the sandpit, the pond, hitting a big rock or a tree and sending him flying from the rear bed to ultimate death. I think we were going about seven miles an hour.

Let the good times roll!

"What's wrong with being a little caution?" he yelled when we returned home from our ride.

"Cautious, it's cautious."

"Yeah, what's wrong with that? It's better to be over caution. I saw that on CNN."

Oh Virgin Mary, that's all I needed— Jake tuning in to current events. The last time he'd insisted on sitting with me as I watched the news, he'd become unglued by the little scroll at the bottom of the screen on reading this little tidbit:

★★Scientists baffled by mysterious acorn shortage★★

It scrolled across the screen twice before the broadcast was interrupted by breaking news: Britney Spears was being wheeled out of her home on a gurney—and the media quite promptly *lost their shit*!

"What about the acorns? What happened to the acorns?" Jake was near hysteria, flipping from channel to channel, trying to get to the bottom of the vague acorn reference. But every channel was reporting on the many facets of the latest celebrity to become a tired mess, rendering the entire body of the American population held captive by pop culture at its lowest ebb.

Screw the squirrels! Brit's gone schitz!

"Mom, what's wrong with that girl? Is she going to die?"

"No."

"Is she sick?"

"Not . . . exactly."

"Where are they taking her?"

The same place I'm going if you keep asking me questions.

We never found out about the mysterious acorn shortage and the probable effect it would have on the poor squirrels of our fine country. Jake handled the situation in the only way he knew how— by hiding out in his room with his Wii, television blaring the thankfully pop-Diva- free Cartoon Network.

I settled in with a good book and a bowl of popcorn.

The next time he ventured out, he held a pencil about six inches from my face and asked, "Can a spell be put on this to make it evil?"

I now know that a piece of popcorn can firmly wedge itself somewhere in the recesses of the nose, taking more than a few moments of pure hell to get out. What you have to do is put a finger to the side of one nostril, close off the opening, and blow out the other nostril. It takes a while and it's not a comfortable feeling, but I can safely assure you that it will come out. On a side note, your throat will be sore for a few days. Probably the salt coupled with all that hysterical choking-slash-laughing.

I scraped the rest of the popcorn from the floor, as well as my lap and cleavage, back into the bag and rolled the top, preparing to take it to the trash can, when I realized Jake was still waiting for a response.

"I'm not even going to dignify that with an answer, Jake."

When I returned from the bathroom, having tossed the popcorn and blown my sore nose, he was sitting in my chair, still waiting.

"What does dignify mean?"

"Go look it up. You've got a dictionary."

I knew full well that even with the definition, he wasn't going to be able to piece my response back together and have it mean anything to him. Call me sadistic but what I *did* know was that it would send him back into his room for at least a few minutes—enough time for me to have a nice laugh at his expense without him being there to witness it. And since the popcorn fiasco had interrupted my original guffaws, I still needed to purge.

I guess he gave up on turning his pencil into the devil's handmaiden. Who knows, maybe he became distracted by one of his cartoons but I'd sure as hell like to know which one because his next question was a doozy.

"What's the gross national product?"

I paused for a few seconds, not because I was trying to torture the kid. Surely he'd had enough. But I had no idea how to explain the gross national product and I wasn't in the mood to do a Google search.

"You know what, honey?" I put out my arms, the universal invitation for a hug. He complied, only slightly willingly. "That's a great question to ask your homeroom teacher tomorrow at school."

You call it passing the buck—I call it getting the most out of my tax money. Teachers get paid to answer questions like that, don't they?

I know I don't because if I did I'd be on the *Forbes* top ten richest people list right now instead of picking kernels of corn from between my couch cushions.

September 10, 2008
Note from Jaxson's Teacher

Jaxson continues to adjust well. We missed a bathroom break this morning because we added Jaxson into kindergarten class for snack, recess, and calendar time today—which he did just great—clapped, sang along with rest of class. So after snack, he was on the playground and just pulled his penis out and went to the bathroom right outside in front of everybody. Ms. Chipman was watching and talked to him—he got in a little funk and sat down for a little bit and then went and played.

On the upside, he did generalize out he can pee outside in more than one place.

On the downside, now he knows he can pee in more than one place: outside.

We'll make up a social story about when Jaxson needs to use a bathroom, and read it to him and send a copy home.

Chuckin' Poppie's Ashes

After seeing something particularly disturbing on television, Jake asks me, "Can that really happen? In real life?"

The answer is easy if he's asking if he can use scissors to cut himself into a different shape, like SpongeBob did in one episode. He went from SpongeBob SquarePants to SpongeBob CirclePants–definitely not something you want to try at home, boys and girls.

It becomes dicier when he's seen something on CNN. There's a fine line between explaining Stranger Danger to your kid and having them hear the gruesome details of some whack job molesting children for sport.

But most disconcerting has to be watching your mother suffocate your grandmother in a bowl of green Jell-O.

My little forays into amateur filmmaking might be a bit confusing to my boys.

Before Mom and I started getting professionals to bring our scripts to the screen, we played every role, including actors.

The whole family got involved–the estrogen-producing ones, anyway. Freud would probably have something to say about the fact that in every story, one of us is either mentally or physically tormenting the other.

As I edited the Jell-O scene, Jaxson sat behind me, watching. At one point, he came around to look at me, took my face in both hands and said, "Tha's not nice."

Sure, come to me when you're forty and tell me you don't want to dunk my head in a vat of Jell-O. Till then, no judgment from the Peanut Gallery, thank you very much.

My filming obsession might require a twelve-step program at some point. But for now, those in my sphere will just have to deal with it.

One year, we planned a birthday celebration for Nanna and decided to kill two birds with one stone— scripting an idea for a short film that ended up requiring a bit of improvising.

In case you haven't figured it out by now, not much is sacred in my family.

Nothin' says lovin' like being made the butt of a deliciously inappropriate joke for one's birthday and having it posted on one of the most visited social-networking-slash-video-sharing websites.

It is truly the gift that keeps on giving.

Nanna was seventy-nine at the time and, in retrospect, we could have given her a heart attack. But that's not what we were thinking about when we called the funeral home and inquired about purchasing a cremation urn identical to the one that housed my grandfather's ashes.

Poppie and his prostate cancer had gone the way of the ash two years previously and we were movin' on.

C'est la vie.

No need to wallow in grief— it'll find you again, soon enough. Steep in it for a few seconds—a week, tops.

Then move on.

"Yes, I wonder if you can help me?" said Mom, stifling giggles as I recorded her making the phone call. "I'm looking for a box like the one my father's ashes are in. There's a dove on it. We purchased one from you a while back and we'd like to get another one."

"The eternal dove? It's a wooden box?" The voice on the other end inquired.

"Yep, that's the one. Do you have any in stock? I can come down and pick it up this week."

And we did.

The plan was to pick Nanna up from her mobile home for a sleepover at Mom's house. My aunt would join us, and there would be fun for all. Mom even had a Ouija board we could pull out if things got boring.

Nanna lives in Dora Pines Mobile Home Park— the last pit stop a senior citizen makes before cooling in a morgue freezer. Her fellow trailer dwellers take great pride in their ten by ten patches of lawn—

mowing, edging, planting, and decorating. Not a yard is safe from tacky accoutrement, garden gnomes, American flags and colorful spinnakers that sit dormant most of the time in the breezeless Florida weather.

When my sister Resi and I pulled into Nanna's driveway, we quickly conspired, "Okay, you go in with that camera and I'll stay in the car and film her coming out with this one. We just need you to be the last one out the door so later she'll think we took the box formerly known as Poppie when she sees the other box."

So I sat and waited as my sister went in, under the guise of having to use the bathroom. Resi made sure to be alone in the living room, furiously taping a quick vignette for the faux video as Nanna carried her bag out to the car.

"Hi, Nanna!" I had the camera in front of my face, already filming, while trying to distract her from the fact that her other granddaughter was alone in her house, up to no good.

"Hello, Jen." Nanna smiled and got really close to the lens.

The ride to my mother's house was a long one, mostly because it was full of Nanna talking about her previous sex life with Poppie. Sure, it was funny— but I also had that feeling you get just before you puke— excessive salivating accompanied by dry heaves.

"I'm on my way to eighty, eighty, tickety-tick de boop," Nanna sang, happy to be the featured star for the weekend. She wasn't in on the plan—she just likes mugging for the camera as much as the rest of us do.

"I ain't got my ear in, that's why I'm talking so loud," she informed us, as if we hadn't already caught on. "I better put it in or your mother will scream at me."

Mom and her sister JoAnn constantly griped at Nanna about wearing her hearing aid. They claimed they didn't like to have to yell, but because we're a raucous bunch by nature, we all talk at a decibel level slightly higher than the average family.

It must be a generational thing. Resi and I can't get enough of Nanna and her antics—her daughters, however, don't enjoy it as much, especially when they're in a public place.

I constantly remind my mother that whatever she does to Nanna, I'll be doing to her in a few years, so she'd better watch it.

Familial karma is a bitch and she's got a wicked backhand.

"You're a good driver, Resi. Not that Jennifer isn't. You're a good driver too."

"Thanks, Nan."

Nanna doesn't travel well. She prefers to sit in the back seat where she won't be able to see if the speedometer hits anything over twenty-five miles per hour.

"Your mother scares the hell out of me lately. When we went up to my sister's house, she was going eighty. I almost shit my pants. When I hollered at her she said, 'Ma, be quiet.' I said, 'Yeah, if you hit something I'll be quiet . . . forever.'"

She regaled us with song, changing the words to fit her mood.

"O, Solo Mio, . . . whose ass are you?"

Who doesn't get tickled when their grandparents talk naughty? It's like the senior citizen version of *South Park*.

"*Yes, sir, he's my baby. No sir, can't get nothing, la-da-da-daaaaay.* That's all right, I've got my you-know-what. Oh, God. That's the best piece of ass I've had all my life."

The "you-know-what" was her vibrator. Apparently, Nanna traveled light— a change of clothes, her dog, and a package of spare batteries.

After we arrived and got settled in, we headed to the back porch to sit around chewing the poo while Mom gave Nanna a perm.

The first fifteen minutes of the conversation were all about toilet paper.

My grandmother has preferences, much like her great-grandson, Jake. She likes very soft, pricey toilet paper. Months earlier, she'd been forced out of her trailer due to an impending hurricane and had to stay with my Aunt JoAnn. They fought the entire time about the lack of appropriate toilet tissue.

"That's the guest bathroom, for God's sake!" said Nanna. "It should have good toilet paper. I wiped myself and got shit on my hand."

Next we discussed Nanna's use of self-tanner. She'd put it on five times that day, which was why the creases in her face stood out— orange crevices making a road map that followed the trail of her laugh lines and crow's feet.

Then she returned to the vibrator discussion.

"Whoever has used a vibrator, raise your hand."

"I'm not getting involved in this," Aunt JoAnn said and promptly left to refill her soda. Resi and Mom both admitted to partaking and I admitted I had not.

"Oh, Jen, honey, you don't know what you're missing." Nanna bounced around in her chair, illustrating the supposed effects of vibrator usage. "Your mother gave me mine. Thank you for the vibrator, Susan."

Mom seemed clueless. "I gave you the vibrator?"

"Yeah, when you cleaned out your closet you gave it to me. I didn't know what it was till I took it home and opened it."

My sister narrated from behind the camera as I took a break from filming. "A used vibrator. My mother gives her mother a used vibrator."

"I washed it. You don't think I'd put it up my twat without washing it?"

Mom looked toward the camera. "I don't remember giving her a vibrator."

"It's probably a back massager," Resi choked out from behind the camera.

After the perm, my mother, sister and I hid in the upstairs bathroom with the urn stand-in and hatched our plan. JoAnn wasn't in on it, and in retrospect it might have been a good idea to clue her in. JoAnn is the sensible one. The rest of us mock sensibility.

The next morning, after a nice breakfast, Mom put the wooden box into a small duffel bag and set it at the end of her dock by the lake.

We lured Nanna out onto the dock and Resi held her hand, just in case she got too close to the side. We didn't want her going into the water since she can't swim—killing Nanna on her seventy-ninth birthday wasn't the plan.

Giving her ticker a little jolt was.

My stepfather took me out on the water in a small, aluminum boat, so I had a front row seat from which to film.

As Resi pretended to show Nanna a turtle in the water, Mom snuck around, removed the box from the duffel bag and prepared to toss it into the lake.

Resi feigned confusion, "Mom, what are you doing?"

This got everyone's attention.

"What's that?" Nanna asked.

"I'm gonna throw it in the lake."

JoAnn, seeing the box, and not in on the plan, went for Mom . . .

Here's where the "short film" portion of our little escapade went south.

Mom chucked the box—it landed a mere three feet away from the dock and bobbed in the water.

Nobody said anything for a long time.

"That's not your father," Nana finally said, rolling her eyes.

JoAnn, however, was a bit more gullible.

There was a fair amount of yelling while I laughed from the boat as the camera jerked around, ensuring anyone viewing the video footage later would need a Dramamine or two.

Kind of like the *Blair Witch Project*.

"Okay, now go get the goddamned box," Nanna yelled.

The script had flopped but we were bound and determined to get it right, so after 'fessing up, Nanna and JoAnn decided to play along. I came in off the boat, found another angle and we prepared for take two.

We'd use the footage from the beginning of the scene, up to the yelling, and then we'd improvise, adding more conflict.

All good stories need conflict.

Resi decided it would be funny if someone actually went into the water, and the rest of us decided she should be that person.

Take two.

It didn't occur to me till after Resi had joined the box that the lake was full of snakes and alligators.

"Get out, get out. There's snakes in there. Get out!" I screamed from behind the camera as my sister struggled to grab the side of the dock.

Nanna, fantastic actress that she is, repeated her initial line without prompting, "Now go get the goddamned box!"

"Screw the box, help me up!" Resi reached for Mom's hand.

"Don't pull your mother in now," Nanna said, watching the box bob in the water a few feet away.

Resi worked her own acting muscle. "What the hell were you thinking?"

"I don't know but the box floats better than you," Mom laughed.

Add some editing and cheesy music and, voila—plenty of hits on YouTube.

Nanna got a few presents that weekend, including an urn that matched her husband's, and few memories she wouldn't soon forget.

Chuckin' Other Shit

"Where's Jaxson?" Jake asked, searching the house.

"I don't know. Probably in his room, busy humping his stuffed Dora the Explorer doll."

"Ugh," Jake rolled his eyes and groaned.

Just then, Jax hobbled into my bedroom, undies around his thighs, and into my bathroom. I peeked in to witness him standing on my bathroom counter, bent over and checking his rear end in the mirror over my sink.

"Oh, yuck! He went poo!" Jake yelled after investigating the boys' bathroom.

"Yes, well those three apples he just ate didn't waste any time working their magic, did they?" I went back to folding the mountain of laundry on my bed.

"Mom, he didn't flush!" Jake whined.

"Huh. Well, flush it for him," I suggested.

"No, gross! Come flush it, please!"

Sigh. Come on, man. Can we move on to issues having nothing to do with toileting? I'm ready for another challenge.

As if on cue, Jax rushed past me once again, dirty underwear in his hand, skid mark clearly visible. "Yucky!"

He proceeded back to the boys' bathroom, opened the cabinet under the sink, chucked them in and slammed the door, before heading back into his room.

"Mom!" Jake screamed, now in full panic mode. Un-flushed poop in the toilet plus a soiled pair of underwear under the sink equaled a catastrophe of epic proportions.

Oh, for the love of Pete! Not another stain-obsessed creature in my midst. I'm still dealing with Jake and his hygiene issues. Must we add the younger one to the mix?

I heard one of Jaxson's dresser drawers open, then a bit of shuffling before the sound of it being shoved closed.

"Gotcha. Good job!" Jaxson exclaimed. He exited his room with a clean pair of tighty-whities hugging his cheeks.

Suddenly I had visions of another few years of constant underwear changing and copious amounts of dirty laundry.

My mother once told me about a dream she'd had where she was a dirty cookie sheet and nobody would clean her. My dream equivalent would have to be drowning in a sea of dirty civvies.

Don't most boys just sort of . . . simmer in their own juices?

I was under the impression that male children didn't mind a little grime. Was every mother required to do a load of underwear every two days, or was it just me?

"Mom! Go get his stinky underwear out of the bathroom!" Jake screamed as he ran into his bedroom, slamming the door.

Flush.

Retrieve scat-a-licious undies.

Check.

Around the time Jaxson was two or three, he began a habit that ended with the neighbor at my door. The unamused neighbor lady and I were destined to dislike one another from that moment on.

Now, let me begin by saying I do not blame her. What awaited her every morning as she headed out to her back porch to enjoy her first cup of coffee certainly wasn't pleasant.

There are quite a few things I wouldn't mind waking up to—breakfast in bed, a spotless house, a one-way airplane ticket to New York City . . .

A backyard riddled with dirty Pull-ups filled with crap, you might have noticed, isn't on that list.

I can only imagine what it looked like— her little veggie garden chock full of Jaxson's good tidings—a minefield of human excrement wrapped in decorative containers.

I'd tried to get him started potty training by purchasing the kind of diapers that were one piece so he could pull them on and off all by himself. I figured giving the kid a bit of control over the situation might make him inclined to take care of business.

He seemed to be doing well on the peeing front. He'd remove a wet diaper, chuck it in the trash and go into his room to get a fresh one, happily pulling it on.

What I didn't put together until later was what he was doing with the number two diapers. Each day, when he went outside to play, he'd find a nice, shady corner of the yard, squat and do a bit of groaning before promptly removing the foul mess and chucking it over the privacy fence.

Since I never actually saw him doing it, I assumed he was putting them in the trash with the others. Never in my wildest imaginings did I think I needed to count the diapers in the trash each night and compare them to how many bowel movements he'd taken throughout the day.

If I had, I would have noticed a glaring error in accounting.

When I opened the door that day, it took me a minute to realize the neighbor lady, whom I'd only met once, had a box full of dirty diapers in her arms.

My first clue should have been her wrinkled nose, the distaste clearly evident on her disturbed countenance.

"Hi there," I offered.

She got right to the point, "I was wondering how long this is going to go on?"

She held out the box, and still I was nowhere near putting two and two together.

"Excuse me?"

She dumped the box at my feet. "Do these look familiar to you?"

I looked down about the same time Jaxson ran up behind me and peeked through my legs, staring at the contents of the box.

If he'd been verbal at the time, he might have said "Ca-ca."

It was then that I recognized the things in the box resembled the thing my kid was wearing at the time. A raggedy-looking diaper with a slightly faded cartoon picture on the front.

"Oh, God."

"Yeah. That's the same thing I say every morning." She wasn't giving an inch and, at that point, my embarrassment morphed into horror.

"I'm so sorry. He's . . . um. He's got some issues. I'm really sorry. But the good thing is, he's actually changing his own diaper. I mean, that's got to count for something, doesn't it?" My weak argument baffled even me.

The woman shook her head and walked away, back to her presumably high-functioning home.

Laxative for the Soul

My mother tells me when I was a shy little girl in kindergarten, I wrote a story about a gumball machine—comparing the little round balls of varying colors to people in the world. I'd share the poem with you, but my mother isn't exactly the type of parent who keeps those kinds of things. No little shoebox of priceless memories or scrapbooks full of photos for her. I'm guessing she read it, smiled, then rolled something into the tiny piece of paper and smoked it.

It was the '70s, after all.

I should note that my mother *is* the type of mother who would, years later, wake me with a 3 AM phone call, "I just had the best idea for a porn movie!" What followed was a three-hour trip to a local store the next day, where I was horrified to find the toy dolls made for young girls now look suspiciously like whores. Out of this shopping adventure came a three-page script for a movie that could only be described as Barbie-Porn—which would, as you will learn, come back to bite me in the ass years later.

Sometime after the gumball poem but prior to the porn, I was a ten-year-old Catholic school girl. Each week we were required to check something out from the library, making sure to carry the book to every class in case we had free time that period. We *had* to read it, as Sister Eugenia would occasionally give us a pop quiz and, unfortunately, this particular nun was familiar with the entire collection in the small library.

I checked out the *The Diary of Anne Frank*. It made a huge impact on me because I related to her. I was about her age. I could *be* her. I could rage against the horrors of a life lived in secret. I, too, could be remembered long after I was gone.

I asked for and was given a diary. My entries were decidedly less awe inspiring than Anne's.

July 9, 1978
Dear Diary,
We went on vacation and it was nice, except there was a strange smell in the VW van the entire trip from something Mom and Dad were smoking. She said they were 'herbs.'
At the Grand Canyon, I was surprised that the railing to keep you from falling was so small. Resi ran right up and swung from it, but I stayed back. I don't know why but suddenly I thought one of my family members might push me over the edge. Could that happen? I don't think any of them are *that* crazy, but the idea would not leave my head, so I stayed back while they all looked.
(p.s. I do not trust them.)
Then we went back to the campground and while Mom and Dad took a nap, Resi and I played with two brothers named Nick and Roger. Roger asked me if I knew what a blow job was.

July 12, 1978
My parents are horrible, horrible people. I must be adopted!!! Resi asked Dad what a blow job was and he said, "What the hell?" and his face got all red and he pulled the VW van over and got out. I hid under my pillow in the back seat and cried, so Mom told me and Resi what it was. My parents are gross!! She said when two people love each other, they do certain things. I said, "Gross things . . . " and she said, "Come back and tell me how you feel about it when you're thirty." I told her she was going to hell and so was Dad. Resi just asked if she brushed her teeth after. My sister is so stupid. I hate my family!!! And I am stuck in this van with them for three more days.

Then came high school and a plethora of unmemorable material which could only qualify as melodrama. Sappy, unrequited love story type of stuff that now would cause my lunch to take a sudden u-turn. I am often reminded of that writing when I talk to my Nanna because she's always watching something or other on Lifetime Television for Women.

Next came the dark period. I cannot recall what these stories were about either, except to say that after reading some of them, my father had one comment. "Jennifer, must everything you write be so . . . maudlin?"

I had to look up maudlin, and thus began another unfortunate chapter in my writing life. My obsession with the dictionary and thesaurus . . .

. . . which spawned my poetry phase. In my defense, I thought everything was *supposed* to rhyme. I'd love to share an example of that early poetry, but at some point I trashed it all so there would be no physical trace of my poetical ineptitude. I think that was around the time we studied Watergate in school.

As I matured, I began paying attention to the world around me. I started to *listen*. This is where my interest in characters developed. Stories do not move me as much as the people in them do. How they speak, what they say, what they aren't saying. I became obsessed with the news, memorizing banter and rewriting it in my head, in an effort to make it more entertaining.

... BREAKING NEWS ...

"I'm Wolf Blitzer and you're here in the CNN newsroom where we've got breaking news to report. We are getting information that a young girl has fallen into the basin of the Grand Canyon. As you can see on our live feed, there is a helicopter flying over the site and our own Anderson Cooper is at the scene. Anderson, what you are seeing?"

"Yeah, Wolf, I'm here in Arizona and if you look behind me you'll see . . . well the side of a building, actually. We are some seven miles from where a young girl has apparently fallen five thousand feet below the rim, into the basin of the canyon. Canyon View Information Plaza is the parks' visitor facility where the press has been cordoned off and we are awaiting news from the recovery teams."

"What a horrible, horrible tragedy. Anderson, thanks for that . . . Now we've got our own Sanjay Gupta, another member of the best news team on television, to help us with this. Sanjay, what can you tell us about a body that might fall some five thousand feet? What kinds of injuries would we expect to find?"

"Well, Wolf, with a fall from that distance, the better question is what injuries wouldn't we expect to find. If you look at this mock-up I've got here, you'll see that the skull, which protects the human brain, is not made to withstand a fall of this kind. It is probably safe to assume this is a recovery effort, at best. What they'll be looking for are small pieces, rather than large ones. Think of a watermelon falling from a ninety-story building and you'll get a clearer idea of what we're dealing with here. On a positive note, it's likely somewhere after falling but prior to landing, one would have a heart attack. Death would be quick . . . in either case."

"Painless?"

"Yes, Wolf, I'd say instantaneous."

"Thanks, Sanjay. Sanjay Gupta, MD. And now we turn to Rob Marciano with a look at the weather these recovery teams will be dealing with. Rob, how's it looking out there?"

"Wolf, unfortunately Mother Nature is brewing up a nasty storm directly over the Grand Canyon right now. So, whatever they're scraping up from that basin, they'd better make it quick. Storms in this area don't usually spur tornadoes, so this will be one for the record books, folks. I don't think I have to tell you what a mess it could be. Think of the large cylinder of wind and rain dipping into that basin and churning the whole canyon bed into something that might resemble the contents of a Cuisinart. Messy, messy stuff . . . Wolf?"

"Just a bad, bad situation. Thanks Rob. Rob Marciano, CNN meteorologist. At the top of the hour we'll join Lou Dobbs, what have you got for us tonight, Lou?"

Then came my Victorian Era. Nudged on by the writings of Oscar Wilde, I wanted to be someone who could describe the fetid contents of a backed-up community toilet with a sophistication and wit that would make it archly amusing.

> *. . . for what is a sophisticated artiste to do*
> *when he stumbles upon an un-flushed loo?*

no verbal riposte or clever bon mot
can resolve such a blunder as a left-sullied pot

What followed was a great deal of reading—everything that the library had to offer from Mr. Wilde. To this day, I cannot get through *The Ballad of Reading Goal* without crying. I think the ironic line spoken by one of his Dorian Gray characters, Lord Henry Wotton, "the less said about life's sores, the better," actually made me the writer I can't help being today.

I gorged on the plays of Edward Albee, the humor of David Sedaris and Augusten Burroughs, the scathing honesty of Chuck Palahnuik and John Rechy—realizing that the further out of the box the fearless author jumped, the more excited I became.

I write because I fancy myself more than just a mother, daughter, wife, or citizen of the world. I have a burning desire to be recognized as something other than eternal caretaker, frantic fixer of boo-boos and chief cook (or defroster) and bottle (or kid) washer.

But mainly, I write to laugh at the ridiculous. Writing, for me, is an emotional laxative, saving me from an impacted soul.

Why ?
by Jake Lopez

Why are pencils #2?
Why are there paperclips?
Why is paper white?
Why is the sky blue?
Why are bananas yellow?
Why is the school made out of brick?
Why do scissors cut?
Why is the number 20, 20?
Why are there pens?
Why do people wear boring gray stuff?
Why do some people hate tubs?
Why is there a brown cow?
Why do cows make milk?
Why do coconuts have milk inside?
Why are there fancy plates?
Why is nature peaceful?
Why are there crowds?
Why do people use curtains?
Why do chickens lay eggs?
Why is there meat?

I Wish I Were Engulfed
in Flames

It was a dark and stormy day.

A bad day. No, really. I mean *bad*. All in all I wish I hadn't been there. A day where, for a brief but very clear moment, I wished I were engulfed in flames. Sweet, searing pain, and then death.

Hail Mary, full of grace. Is there a flamethrower in the vicinity?

And then I heard it, amid the cacophony of screams inside my head and out.

"Is there anything I can do . . . to help?"

That day, I met an angel at the Rite Aid drugstore, and immediately thought of Blanche Dubois and relying on the kindness of strangers. My child was in the middle of a full-on hysteria-inducing temper tantrum because I would not purchase him another camera to replace the one he'd put into the toilet and flushed the night before.

The toilet was unscathed—the camera, however, hadn't been so lucky.

I'd stopped at the drugstore to pick up a new prescription for Jaxson, the third in a series of medications to try and help prevent his aggressive behavior, particularly at school. See, they kind of frown on biting, hitting, and throwing things when there are other children around who might be in harm's way. That I can understand. If I had a "normal" child, I wouldn't want another kid around mine who might kick them. In fact, I'd be heading up the parade to chuck that kid out of school by his Underoos.

But because I'm not the beneficiary of one of those children, I can only hope the other parents understand the need for my children to be included in the same classes and activities as theirs. I further hope that these parents would understand that when they send their precious cherubs out into the real world, there's a very good chance that they'll, at some point, be working or interacting with someone who might have a disability—in which case, it's probably a good idea to start them on the road to acceptance and education now, rather than when any sort of prejudice and ignorance have been engrained too deeply to be corrected. Like racism and homophobia, those kinds of roots are planted pretty deep.

This goes for the general public, as well.

When I am in the grocery store and my child suddenly rolls into tantrum mode, kicking and screaming and such, it's not very helpful if passersby say things like, "He needs a good spanking," or "You wouldn't see my kid acting like that."

I have stock replies to these uneducated and blatantly rude statements, but often it takes something different to get my point across. I like to pass my child to them over the deli meats and say, "Go ahead, hit him. Let's see if it works." And then I take a seat on the cold tile floor, lean over, and let my forehead benefit from the temperature and wait it out. This accomplishes two things. I get a much needed break, and the offender in question gets embarrassed as they try to decide what to do with the kid presently sinking his teeth into their shoulder.

Eventually I sit up and tell them that I am tired, and not above leaving the store immediately— alone . . . and forever. Generally, at about that time, they think I'm crazier than the kid they're holding and often look a little frightened as I stand up and begin to back away, waving to my son.

"Bye, honey. This nice man is gonna take you home. Have fun . . ."

Okay, so I don't *actually* do this. But I *really, really* want to.

Usually I tell them that a little autism education might be in order, and say it in a way—because I am a writer and good with words— that makes them feel like the pile of dirt they are. Sometimes I top it off with a general observation about their attire, weight, or lack of front teeth.

Okay, so I don't do that either because I am the better person.

Really, do people think it's helpful to the parent in question to make derisive comments at the same time their child is pulling down a display in the automotive section? I always want to ask but at moments like those, I'm usually in a flop sweat, nursing a couple of painful bites, feeling certain my heart is beating fast enough that a heart attack or stroke is imminent, and frankly, I'm really not in the mood. God help you if I'm on the rag because then things are liable to get ugly.

Go ahead, make my day.

When dealing with a certain type—an overly coiffed, fully made up female with a cell phone to her ear, an air of entitlement mingling in the wake of her pricey but asthma-inducing perfume—I have to admit, I might take a little too much pleasure. A snide comment or a look of disdain in this instance would not behoove her. Jake can be made to vomit on site if any number of topics are broached in his presence. So the next time you're standing in line behind me as my child is wailing, pulling items off the impulse racks, and you feel the need to tell the person on the other end of the line that you're "... behind some woman who can't control her kids ...," you might want to take a few steps back.

"Jake? Did you like dinner last night? It was sautéed cockroaches and rat droppings. *Mmmmmm.* Wasn't it good?"

It will happen pretty quickly and I'm not above using my own kid to prove a point.

"Yeah, that's probably gonna stain because he drank Hawaiian punch earlier and that stuff has got more red dye #4 in it than is safe for human consumption."

And then I smile.

But on the particular day in question, I'd bent over, grabbed Jaxson like a sack of potatoes, tossed him over my shoulder, and proceeded to make my way out of Rite Aid as he pummeled me from behind, sinking his teeth into my arm. My purchases fell from the plastic bag, trailing behind me like Hansel and Gretel's breadcrumbs.

Then, the angel appeared.

Without asking, without my silent pleading eyes meeting hers, she quietly followed me to the parking lot, picking up my prescriptions, hair spray, box of tampons and bag of Hershey's kisses, gathering them all up as I maneuvered to press Jaxson against the car with my body, fishing for my keys.

It took ten minutes to unlock the door and push my screaming child inside. I closed the door and stood outside the car for a moment, taking a look at the nice bruise on my arm that was already forming, his little teeth imprints clearly in the center. She handed me the bag and smiled as Jaxson wailed inside the car, banging on the window, his voice only slightly muffled by the closed windows.

"Here you go."

"He's autistic," was the only thing I could think of saying. What I wanted to say was, *Please take me home with you. I can't handle this for one more second.*

"Yeah, I kind of guessed there was something going on there besides the regular old tantrum. Can you get home okay?"

Will you marry me? I wanted to kiss her on the mouth. Right there in the parking lot. I wanted to drown out the howling in the car behind me with some other, more pleasant sensation.

My eyes filled with tears and I shook her hand. "Thanks. You have no idea how nice it is to have someone not judging me right now."

"I think I can guess." She smiled, touched my arm gently and then quietly proceeded to her car.

Why I Hate Pokemon

Jake wrote a letter to the Pokemon Headquarters with his handwritten instructions and a detailed schematic for what he called the Pokemon Worldwide, an invention he was sure they could whip up for him.

I, in turn, mailed it after enclosing a letter of my own— checking yet another thing off my to do list, as well as my conscience.

Dear Sirs,

Forgive my intrusion, but I thought I'd tuck this letter into the envelope my son Jake was sending, in an effort to explain his query a bit.

Jake is a 12-year-old autistic boy, and from a very young age, he's been obsessed with all things Pokemon.

For the last few years, he's become preoccupied with the idea that a sort of "Pokemon World" could be created whereby Pokemon characters could be released into the real world via a sort of reverse ATM machine.

Well, you and I both know this isn't possible and I've spent the better part of the last few years doing my best to explain this to him, through various ways and means, with much stress to my already teetering sanity.

When he was seven, he sent a letter to Santa (about five years ago, actually) asking for this machine and I had to "send" a letter back from Santa, in an effort to try and buy some time until he reached an age where he'd understand the impossibility of what he was asking.

I'll enclose the Santa letter, as well as a documentary on *dvd* that I've produced, called *every journey is unique: a tale of autism*. In this, you can see how he reacted to the letter, as well as a few other things relating to his video games and Pokemon.

But, the basic reason I'm writing this and secretly putting my letter into his envelope before it gets sent, is that it would be *extremely helpful* to me if you could respond with a letter—something written on professional "Pokemon" letterhead—something that could gently let him down in a way that a mother cannot.

Come on, take one for the team. And by team, I mean me. Make something up— I really couldn't care less at this point, but I'd like to move forward and not have to discuss Pokemon on a daily basis.

Pokemon is ruining my life.

Even though Jake now knows the truth about Santa Claus, he still believes some scientist somewhere can create this "Pokemon Worldwide" he envisions.

As a parent, I don't want to shatter his dreams, but have no problem asking you to do it, since I've spent my fair share of money on your products.

As I said, a simple letter on official-looking company stationery would probably do it.

Thanks in advance for the time and attention,
Desperate Mother in Michigan!

P.S. Attached is the response "Santa" left for Jake on Christmas Day.

Dear Jake,

I received your letter and understand you wish to have something called *Pokemon Worldwide*, so you can make Pokemon come to life . . .

I am trying to invent this new toy, but it takes *years* to create a new toy, as we here at the *North Pole* take great care in making each toy *perfect*.

I hope you will understand and be patient.

We have already begun construction on this *Pokemon Worldwide*, but there have been some problems, like Pikachu jumping out the size of the Empire State building. I'm sure you understand that wouldn't be good for anyone.

As soon as we complete the prototype *Pokemon Worldwide*, you are on a list to be the *first* to receive one, but again, *please be patient*.

Estimated time of completion of this new and fantastic toy: *October, 2015*

Please enjoy the other toys I've brought you, and don't be too disappointed, as the *elves* are hard at work on the *Pokemon Worldwide*. . . . in fact Elf #357, Conrad, just got hit by a flying spit wad that *Kyogre* tried to shoot at *Groudon*, and another problem has arisen, as both of these Pokemon came out of the *Pokemon Worldwide prototype* smelling like poop. (We can't have that can we?)

Merry Christmas, Jake!

Love

Santa Claus

    Of course, I heard nothing in response, which might have had something to do with the fact that I alluded to the fact—okay I specifically said—that Pokemon was ruining my life.
    I guess not everyone finds honesty as refreshing as I do.

I put in the smelly poop reference, hoping to dissuade Jake from his game fetish— he doesn't like the topic of poop, or anything even remotely related to it.

As a friend pointed out, she couldn't think of a better way to illustrate for my son that the cartoon game character he so revered was, indeed, full of shit.

Full Renal Failure

Renal sounds like anal, doesn't it? I'm ashamed to say pondering the similarities gives me the giggles—and anal failure is quite a bit funnier anyway.

There's nothing like the possibility of a terminal illness to harsh your mellow. At this point, my Catholic upbringing won't even allow me the modest fantasy life I once permitted myself to wallow in. I don't deserve it—I am a horrible, selfish person. I do not need anyone else to point this fact out to me. It's as plain as the corpulent puss oozing from a bedsore that I will one day have because there will be nobody to take care of me but the nursing home worker who is paid minimum wage to do so.

My husband has kidney "issues." Up to this point, the fact never occurred to me that the breadwinner in my household could become disabled, requiring constant care. I've already got two autistic children. Exactly how much am I expected to take before I'm allowed a nervous breakdown? Who do I call to complain to and am I going to incur long distance charges? I need specifics—something in writing, if possible.

It seems like the bitch-slap of fate or just karma. Whoever is up there taking notes has quite the ironic sense of humor, and I don't appreciate sardonic wit when I'm scared. In fact, I could probably be described as being paralyzed with fear, if the option were even available to me. It isn't. I still have to make school lunches, do homework, prepare dinner, wash dishes, and keep some clean laundry around the house. I could actually kill myself for ever complaining about such trivial things as taking out the trash. Today, I'd be happy to clean the toilets if I didn't have the added burden of possible death hovering over me, crushing any hope of normalcy.

I've always labored under the presumption that all one had to do to live a decent, protected life was to be an unselfish person, treat others as you'd have them treat you, do the occasional bit of volunteer work, and pay your taxes. Clearly this isn't the case. I don't mean to sound ungrateful, but at this point, I'm feeling a bit like a bird being battered by the frigid February winds so common here in Michigan— more than a bit cold and blown around by life's natural disasters.

First came the swelling—fluid-filled ankles that resembled sausages stuffed into glossy, tight skin. Next came the headaches, ones he rarely complained about, another warning sign that went undetected because of his inability to admit to any physical discomfort.

Then there was the back pain. Deep, throbbing lower backache that made it impossible for him to find a comfortable position, whether lying down or standing. It breaks you to see someone you care about feeling badly, never mind being in pain.

Renal + failure = pertaining to the kidneys and the lack of success related to them.

So, basically my husband has unsuccessful kidneys. Kidneys that pass blood and protein. Apparently that's not good. People need their kidneys in proper working order and his are causing his blood pressure and cholesterol levels to skyrocket. Another host of issues that, in and of themselves, can cause possible death. I don't really want to know how bad it can get, and he hasn't even been diagnosed yet.

Two days ago, he went for a needle biopsy. As I sat in the chair awaiting his return to the little cubicle, I was forced to listen, for six long hours, to the woman across the hall. She was also undergoing a needle biopsy, hers on the liver. Clearly, she wasn't concerned. I know this because she kept saying she wasn't concerned. She ordered a turkey sandwich from Subway—lettuce, hot peppers, green peppers and red onions, a large diet soda and a cookie. And when her friend went to fetch them for her, she proceeded to make a series of cell phone calls to friends and family, outlining the extent of her concern, or lack thereof. I also learned that her husband Mike would be there in two hours to pick her up, straight from a court appearance, whereby he was sentenced to fourteen days in jail, for what I'm not sure. But as far as she was concerned, he got off easy. It could have been a year in jail. Third offense.

Then she called someone named Brad, who seemed to be a work colleague, though I couldn't be sure because there was a fair amount of flirtatious banter going on. I wanted to hurl my husband's size 9 work boot through the flimsy cubicle curtain and have it land somewhere around her right temple.

I didn't know this woman, but I knew I didn't like her. Probably because when her friend came back with her six-inch Subway sandwich, they proceeded to eat while watching CNN, and at some point the woman, who had now repeated twelve times that she was not concerned about her needle biopsy, commented on how Newt Gingrich would be a great presidential nominee in 2012.

Barak Obama was barely one hundred days into his presidency and she had the audacity to be thinking about the next election and, God forbid, another Republican in the White House.

Maybe that's the definition of anal failure.

I don't consider myself to be exclusionary. I don't care who you have sex with, pray to, or what color skin you happen to have been born with. I do, however, have a violent distaste for conservative extremists. And anyone that works at FOX News—and that's playing it fast and loose with the word "news"—or watches that particular television channel. As far as I'm concerned, Ann Coulter can rot in hell alongside Bill O'Reilly and Rush Limbaugh. And as long as they aren't allowed to reproduce behind the gates of Hades, I'm happy to forget them altogether.

At this point I tried my best to tune her out, burying my nose in the latest Augusten Burroughs novel. I tried, I really did. But the constant blathering continued— she barely took a breath between bites. I could hear the Baked Lays Chips crunching, and the slurping sound her Diet Coke made traveling its way up the straw and past her Botoxed lips. I recognized the acidic rise of impending homicidal behavior travel up my esophagus like bile. Surely I was on the brink of multiple psychotic episodes.

How dare she enjoy her sub sandwich when my husband was having a needle thrust through his skin, into his kidney? How dare she be unconcerned about her own liver, to the point that she had the presence of mind to make a business call and eat crappy take-out?

"Yep, we'll get on it right away," she says through her mouthful of sub. "Substitute the D-17 model for the D-14. No problem. Thanks so much. We'll talk soon."

When they bring my husband back into the cubicle, he seems to be in the same condition as when they took him in: slightly uncomfortable from the back pain, but none the worse for wear.

Then begins a six-hour wait. Before they release him, they must be sure there is no internal bleeding. Blood pressure checks every half hour. He has to lie flat for the first two hours, something that is difficult at best. But he soldiers through like a good boy, hardly complaining as I play the part of comic relief.

I hold his penis as he attempts to pee into the small "bucket" they've given him so they can monitor his urine. He grabs my ass playfully as I hold the urinal while he fills it. We both pretend this is just another day, just another place to cop a feel. But we know it's not true. I rarely touch him anymore. We rarely communicate on a physical level and that knowledge alone smacks of desperation.

We laugh silently, mocking the woman in the cubicle across from us. In fact, she's just about to get out of the bed and head to the bathroom when a nurse intervenes, telling her that she, too, is the unwilling recipient of six hours of lying on her back. She does, in fact, say her back hurts a bit.

Good, I want to scream, *take a nap and spare the rest of the short-stay ward another of your lengthy cell phone calls.*

I flash my husband a bare breast and he smiles, grabbing for it as well as any patient who's just had a two-inch needle piercing their kidney can. Then we laugh at the fact that his bottle of piss is sitting next to his hospital lunch. It looks like beer, an inch of foam floating above the yellow liquid. I pretend to toss it across the cubical at our jabber-jawed Republican neighbor. A little sloshes out and his immediate look of panic sets me into a silent fit of giggles, though his laughter seems to be causing him a bit of discomfort so I settle back down into my uncomfortable chair.

Four hours into his forced bed rest, I thank God the movie *Twister* is being shown on the hospital television. Anything to keep his attention for a few minutes and allow me a break from playing Jim Carrey. It's just too exhausting.

When the nurse enters and tells us he can go, that his blood work didn't identify any internal bleeding, I sigh audibly, then try to cover my concern by burping. She leaves and he hops too quickly out of the bed, wincing in pain. I think he might faint. I am not used to this physical disrepair. He's a strong man, or he used to be. I've seen him lift a couch by himself, and more than once he'd flipped our oversized king mattresses for me with ease. Now he can barely lower himself into the wheelchair to be pushed downstairs as I hurry to bring the car around to the front of the building. Thank God the orderly won't let him out of his sight till I'm behind the wheel because he still thinks he's driving the hour and a half home.

I tell him today I'm the chauffeur and stifle the urge to laugh out loud at the image of Morgan Freeman and Jessica Tandy in *Driving Miss Daisy*.

In my head, it's the hysterical laughter of the insane ricocheting off my skull.

Zeitgeist: Reality

I hate reality shows. In fact, putting the words *reality* and *television* together is oxymoronic. I've told Jake, because Jaxson's still too young to get the concept, that nothing that emanates from that square box in the living room *or* the other square boxes in each of the bedrooms—because with autistic thinkers you need to be specific—none of it is real. So now, basically he thinks Anderson Cooper is as fake as Elmo.

Works for me.

I just don't understand the concept of reality television. Maybe I'm missing something here, and the Lord in Heaven above knows there's enough fodder in my life to cover at least five seasons of a new reality show, but what's the point? I don't need an editor culling my life into embarrassing tidbits for the world to salivate over. I have no problem making myself look like an idiot all on my own.

I don't so much mind the reality programming that involves actual skill like *Project Runway* or that show where they groom dogs. And I enjoy the heck out of that one where they pit chefs against one another. Let the sashimi fly. But when it involves children, I just don't understand the inclination. If I want to exploit my children, I'll do it on my own time so America can't see the unsightly piles of laundry and unwashed dishes. Like in a book, under the guise of educating the general public about autism.

Everyone remember little Falcon, the kid we all originally thought had climbed into a homemade balloon aircraft in Colorado and floated away? That high-speed land and foot chase as cops followed the silver space ship until it hit the ground, only to find it empty?

Before the rest of America and I realized it was all a hoax by a family with reality show envy, I actually believed it to be true. My first thought was this:

MISTAKE NUMBER ONE: Parents of two boys leaving a balloon contraption tethered in the backyard. That's like a sign from God to a kid: "Here, jump in and take a ride!"

But it was easy to see how it *could* have happened.

Once upon a time, my husband left a ladder up against the house we lived in that had a low, flat roof. We'd been doing interior construction.

The next day, about the time I'd applied vibrant red hair color to my hair and stepped out to the back porch to check on my little one, who was four at the time, I realized I hadn't seen him in approximately five minutes. I knew he couldn't get out of the back yard where he'd been playing because we had an eight-foot-high privacy fence around the perimeter and the front door was dead-bolted at the door frame because he's autistic and prone to The Great Escape.

In a panic, I unlocked the door anyway, probably assuming he'd somehow flown over the fence—hell, I didn't know *what* had happened, but the terror that settled into my bowels for the next three minutes is, even now, indescribable.

See, he wasn't verbal at the time. He cooed and grunted and made noises but if he were lost, he couldn't even respond to his own name.

So there I was in my hair coloring outfit—a tube dress thing that barely covered my underwear, and I'm screaming and running around the front yard, yelling Jaxson's name. Cars flew by the busy intersection, possibly entertained by the half-naked woman with flaming red goo now dripping down her face. But nobody stopped.

Then I heard it. A sound like a bird chirping, or a small animal cooing. I followed the sound, my heart beating out of my barely covered chest, boobies dangerously close to escaping, and spotted Jaxson on the roof. He was playing with the tiny rocks that had been put there by the roofers, mesmerized as a handful slid between his fingers into his lap.

Now the dilemma. If I ran back to the front yard, through the house and around back, would he fall from the roof, his head exploding on the cement like a ripe melon tumbling off the back of a vegetable truck?

No, I couldn't risk it. So I did the next best thing. I climbed atop the front of my husband's prized 1969 MGB Midget and heard it dent under my feet as I reached up, barely able to grab his little hand as he laughed and fell forward into my arms.

About the same time my tank top slid off my breasts. Anyone passing the corner of First and Simpson streets that day got an eyeful, that's for sure.

I hugged Jaxson to me, his little body covering my nakedness and cried as I ran into the house, not giving a moment of thought to the car I'd probably just ruined.

Later that night, when I relayed this story to my husband, he appeared to be more concerned about the condition of the car than the possible death of our child. I remember mumbling something about a misplaced ladder, the possibility of divorce, and his impending death and dismemberment.

If there had been a television crew in the vicinity, a whole lot of bleeping would have been necessary in post-production. Hell hath no fury like a woman whose own reality show has come perilously close to being permanently canceled.

Thumb Tack
by Jake Lopez

People all over the world buy thumb tacks.
They are important.
I like thumb tacks very much.
They are useful.
I play with one.
Thumb tacks are great.

Oprah's the Reason My Kid Thinks I Want to Drown Him in the Tub

When Jake was five, he slid into the living room as I stood in the adjoining kitchen over a boiling pot, tie-dyeing a set of curtains. Oprah was on the television and Jake's sneakers squeaked against the wooden floor as he skidded to a stop just after hearing this: "We're here with Rusty Yates, husband of Andrea Yates, the woman who, as we all know by now, drowned her five children in the bathtub."

He did that slow-look-over-his-shoulder thing the pursued victim in a horror movie does just before someone hacks them into fifteen hundred pieces.

I knew, at that moment, I was screwed.

"Who is that? Who drowned her children?"

I turned the burner off under the pot and sunk into a kitchen chair.

Why, Lord? Why me? Truly. Have I committed some karmic malfeasance this week, or was I a phone solicitor in some former life, and am now being repaid for torturing people with bad credit to their ultimate suicides?

"Honey. You know how you get sick? Like with a cold? Or when your cousin Priscilla broke her arm? Well this lady was sick, but in her head. It's not something you can catch like the flu. But she did something very, very bad and she'll go to jail for it."

"Were the kids being bad?"

Oh man. My heart broke a little that day when I saw the fear in his eyes. The idea that a child could think they could ever do something so bad that their parent would drown them in a tub was almost too much for me to bear.

"No, honey. Of course not. There was something wrong with her. She did something bad, not the children. Now they're in heaven with God."

Screw you, God. Screw you, *and* Oprah, and *me* for even having the damned television on because it seems to be a hotbed for breeding fear and we won't even start on the self-loathing it creates because there aren't enough hours in the day.

I grabbed the remote and clicked off the television, motioning for Jake to sit on my lap.

"Sweetie, some people are just sick in their brains and that makes them do very bad things. But those people get caught and go to jail so you don't have to worry, okay?" I knew I was lying to him and it made me physically ill. Not every sicko gets caught and goes to jail, but I'd rather chop off my left arm than have my autistic child worry about even one more thing in addition to everything else he had to deal with on a daily basis.

He stared at the blank television screen for long moments before getting off my lap and going to forage in the refrigerator for something to drink.

I watched him for a minute and when he didn't inquire further, I figured I was off the hook. Sometimes it was like that. Interest waned— the kid had the attention span of a gnat sometimes, while other times he could obsess about something until you were praying for sweet relief in the form of an impending tornado.

Good. Now I could rinse my newly tie-dyed curtains, put them in the dryer and get dinner started.

I began to pry open the container of barely-thawed ground beef as he sipped his juice box.

"Okay, I'm gonna make spaghetti for dinner. Go take your bath and I'll be in there to wash your hair in a minute."

Jake slurped the last of his juice, tossed it into the trash and was almost out of the kitchen when he stopped suddenly in his tracks. That slow look over the shoulder was even more ominous the second time around, and immediately I realized my mistake.

The meat-sickle landed on my toe, but I barely registered the pain as I hurried over to him, this time unable to control my tears. I hugged him tightly as I cried.

"Honey, listen to me. There is *nothing* you could ever do to make me drown you in the bathtub, do you understand? *Nothing.* There is nothing that would ever make me that mad or sick or—"

"—are you sure?"

"Yes, positive."

"What if *I* killed someone, then would you be mad?" the five-year-old asked.

I pulled him away from my chest and looked him in the eyes, smiling, "Are you planning on killing someone?"

"No."

"Okay, then we're good." I gave him a tap on the backside and nudged him toward the bathroom. "I love you, buddy."

"I know," he said, hopping toward the bathroom.

When he was younger, that's how he always responded to me telling him I loved him. Now he initiates it, telling me he loves me at least seventeen times a day, probably out of a sense of insecurity. But back then, I said it first and he said, *I know.* But I cherish every one of those *I knows* because unlike reminding me that he loves me over and over out of compulsion, then he was simply and very literally responding to what I'd said.

Knowing that *he* knew was a greater gift than I could ever have hoped for.

I heard the bath water turn on as I bent to pick the meat up from the floor, rinsing it in the sink, and tossing it back into the pan with a metallic thump.

What were a few floor germs compared to the thought of impending death by bathtub drowning, right?

The Rule: Drink Your Milk
by Jake Lopez

The reason people should drink their milk is because it is healthy.
Milk is a dairy product.
The milk at school is HORRIBLE!
I like the milk at home better than the very boring school milk.
People should always drink milk at home and never at stupid school.
There are all kinds of milk.
Well, not a lot: There is cow milk and goat milk.
The worst place to drink milk is the boring, stupid school.
I think school milk can make people have a disease.
So you should never drink school milk unless you want to get a disease.
The milk you drink at home is 100% healthy.
The school milk is 100% bad for you.
You should always drink healthy milk.

Never a Dull Moment

jlcallmejeni: YOU ARE NOT GOING TO BELIEVE THIS ONE ... LOL

Suesan0814: What?

jlcallmejeni: Ok, so Jax wanted to play on the computer so I pulled out my laptop and downloaded a few of his movies so he could watch. He's having fun watching them and I turn around and he's figured out *how to tape a video using the camera in the frigging laptop.* I didn't even know the laptop had a camera in it. Anyway he's making video clips of himself and watching them.

Suesan0814: Holy shit!

jlcallmejeni: I never even knew how to do it! And I'm all dumb coming up behind him, "Hey, what are you doing? *Oh* look you're on the computer screen. Hey, wait, are you recording this?!"

Suesan0814: Oh God tomorrow he'll probably have his own v-log! Well, let's hope he doesn't try to take it into the tub with him.

jlcallmejeni: Meanwhile, you know that fetish site I joined yesterday to research for Wisdom? Now I've got an email titled 'Welcome to Fet Net' in my inbox from someone named Brutus Maximus.

Suesan0814: Hahahahahaha never a dull moment.

I am certain I've been put on some watch list somewhere. The contents of my hard drive contain research on everything from autism, to how to dispose of a body, to zoophilia— and there are some interesting sites about Dubya Bush in there as well. I'm guessing an incorrect correlation has been made by Big Brother and I expect a visit from the FBI any day now. In preparation, I make sure I'm wearing my best undies and there's fresh lemonade in the refrigerator. I know a little something about being a hostess.

I was just clearing the last of my inbox when Jake approached me, yanked down his pants and underwear, bent over and spread his cheeks.

"Mom, can you check my butt and see if I have any poo in it?" the twelve-year-old queried, his hair brushing the carpet as he stared at me upside down from between his legs.

The funny thing is, I didn't even blink. Just part of the job. I struggle to recall what I put on my resume just prior to motherhood that required me checking his bung-hole daily for dingle-berries. I mean, I'm glad he's trying for hygiene and all, really. But I worry over an image of him at college, squatting over his camera, taking a digital picture, and sending it via email so I can check his lower orifice on the Internet. Somewhere along the line we've redefined the word normal. Or dysfunction. I'm not sure which.

I've got such a screwed up family, but it speaks volumes that they all seem perfectly normal to me. My Nanna is the funniest one. She's eighty-four and says anything that comes into her head, believing she's past the age where any sort of edit mode is warranted. Whenever I'm around her, I have to bring the video camera because there's no movie in the world that could fully illustrate the character she is in real life.

Mom went to Florida recently to visit and had to take her to the doctor because she had some sort of rash on her thigh. The first thing Nanna says to Dr. Rodgers is, "Now, I don't have VD. I haven't had a dick near me since the '70s. So what the hell is this shit?"

She calls Neosporin *neo-sperm,* and once announced to a packed theater during a showing of *Gigli* that, "I never liked the sex. Too messy and then you have to douche." Why did you pay good money to go see

Gigli, you might be asking yourself? Nanna picked the movie— that's the only explanation I have because aside from the slightly interesting vagina monologue in the middle, my recollection of the event is that it was one hundred and twenty-one precious minutes of my life I'll never get back.

I'm still concentrating on my email and I don't look into the abyss of Jake's butt but just glance at it peripherally and say, "Looks good to me, buddy."

He groans. "Mom! Look! Please! Is there any poo left?"

I turn my head to the right, stare into his butt hole for a good few seconds and then pull a concerned face.

"What? What is it?" There is panic in his voice.

When I start to laugh, Jake hobbles into my room, his pants and boxers around his ankles. He gives the mirror a try, peeking around the side of his bent body in an effort to get a proper look.

"I was just kidding buddy! You're clean," I yell from the other room as I notice Jaxson has followed his brother into the room and is watching the entire drama unfold.

"Ugh. You're so rude!" Jake yells, pulling up his pants as he heads back to his room.

Yeah, I'm the rude one in this scenario.

Okay, listen. Here's the deal. I have absolutely no problem with my kids' *issues*. If Jake can't poop and then clean himself with toilet paper like everyone else in the free world, and needs baby wipes to complete the task, fine by me. But I believe it's my job as a parent to educate him on the subtleties of life. Like, the average response to someone bending over for an anal examination just might be laughter. I have no problem living with his horror of eccentricities. I do, however, feel I wouldn't be doing my job if I didn't show him, in a way that is meaningful to him, that the responses he's likely to get from said activities might not be conducive to having a normal social life.

And then I see it. A movement from the bedroom. I peek in to witness the dysfunction instantly multiplying. Jaxson is now naked and hovering over the floor above one of my makeup mirrors and is staring into his booty hole. With both knees bent, he bobs up and down, watching his little sphincter pucker open and closed.

Check please . . .

Just let me sign, add a nice tip, and be on my way because at this point I don't think my parenting is doing any good. Not for them, not for me, not for the possible spouses who will have to take over poo-duty one day.

Oh God, the horror. Can you imagine what level of sainthood the person who took on this dog and pony show would be required to display?

Even eating a simple meal with Jake is a nightmare. Mom and I took him to Frisches Big Boy one morning to give him a little outing on his own. The first thing he wanted, no *needed* to do was have his picture taken with the ten-foot-tall Big Boy in the lobby. Forget about the line of people waiting to sidle up to the buffet like hungry cattle, all watching in amused bewilderment— Jake doesn't notice those things. So Mom pops out her cell phone and sets up the shot as snickers and guffaws are directed at the hundred and twenty-pound smiling kid with his arm slung around Big Boy's waist.

The hostess tells us to take a seat, and thankfully, I arrive at the booth first and I'm able to flick the dead fly from the sticky table before Jake sees it, because if he had seen it first, all bets would have been off. Nobody would have been eating that day.

We're no sooner seated with menus in our hands then he starts in.

"Grammy, you're not going to do the teeth thing, right?"

I feel the laughter trying to break free already and see Mom is also struggling to keep it together. "No, Jake, I won't do the teeth thing."

The teeth thing in question is when Mom sucks at one of her teeth when trying to remove food, making a *ttthhhhhttttt* sound that sends him through the roof. For some reason he associates it with the rat "issue" we had in a previous home— that and passing any Auto Zone.

Let me pull it all together for you.

He once availed himself of the lavatory in one of their auto parts stores in Florida and some joker had put a fake rat on the floor in the corner. I found that amusing— Jake thought otherwise. In any event, all discussion of rats, auto parts or that *thhhhhhhttttt* sound can bring on a series of unfortunate events that will ultimately lead to my needing a fistful of Xanax.

On any given day, there are enough land mines to dodge that I often have trouble keeping track. So does Mom, who regularly sucks her teeth in his presence and then has to do something quickly to distract him. It never works. He can't hear me screaming for him across the room when it's time to do homework, but a little teeth sucking must sound like a lawn mower to his sensitive ears.

At any rate, she promised not to suck her teeth, we all ordered, and I nervously awaited the next thing that might happen to sully our breakfast event. And it was an event. For the reasons mentioned above, and many more, we rarely take Jake out to eat. And you can forget about taking Jaxson to a restaurant. That just doesn't happen.

By the time we get our drinks, Mom and I are working really hard to stifle the giggles because when you just know something is going to happen, when you expect it but aren't sure which direction it's going to come from, it's like a sadistic game of Where's Waldo— except Waldo is a meltdown and what you really want to do is kill Waldo.

Jake wipes his nose on a napkin and because Mom and I both know there's not a chance in hell that dirty napkin will be allowed to remain at the table, we immediately start looking around for the nearest trash receptacle. Jake's already on his feet, meandering through the restaurant, in and out of tables, looking back at us and then back around the room, his face becoming increasingly more alarmed.

"Oh Jesus, here we go . . . " Mom mutters, pointing to where she thinks the bathroom might be. We can't see it, but it's the only part of the restaurant, save the kitchen, that we can't see, so we assume it's over there somewhere.

But clearly it's not because Jake's turned back around and headed for us, his eyes wide, the dirty napkin clutched tightly between thumb and forefinger, held straight out from his body like toxic waste.

"I told you we should have just taken him to the McDonalds drive-thru," I mumble just as a busboy wheels his cart past us to clean a nearby table. Mom starts furiously pointing to the little trash hamper attached to his cart and Jake makes a beeline for it, tossing in the napkin.

His world rights itself again for one brief shining moment as he flops back down into his seat.

Then he looks at his hands and grimaces.

The iced tea Mom has just sipped dribbles from her mouth as she laughs out loud, but thankfully she wipes it from the table with her sleeve before Jake can look up again.

"Here . . . " Mom, ever the prepared grandmother, pulls a bottle of antibacterial hand cleaner from her purse and squirts it into Jake's hands right before the waitress arrives with our food.

I think the loud sigh of relief that shoots out of me concerns the waitress, but I just smile and dig into my plate, knowing the expiration date on this little venture out is approaching quickly.

There are a blissful few seconds when all I can hear is the quiet din of other diners conversing and cutlery scraping against plates.

Few is the operative word here.

"Mom, you're not going to eat with your mouth opened, right?"

. . . and the beat goes on . . .

Random Heartbreaking Conversations over Coffee

Some of the saddest conversations I've ever had, I associate with the smell of fresh brewed coffee. Maybe because there's a safety in holding a steaming mug in front of you— the safety of an everyday object. I need some safety in my life, so I'm always holding a cup of coffee.

"Mom, do you think I have a passion for dogs?" Jake sat at the kitchen table as I finished the last of the dishes, waiting for a pot of coffee to percolate.

"Sure I do," I replied, wiping my forehead with the back of my hand.

"But I've made so many mistakes with animals in the past." There was a lifetime of regret in his statement, for good reason.

Visions of dead animals danced through my mind, like sugarplums in the heads of small children on that Holiest of Toy-Filled Eves.

Like the mouse he'd run over— a five-year-old drive-by, his chubby legs pumping the pedals of his tricycle as he followed the little white flash across the carport. He didn't mean to kill the poor thing— he was just racing him to the finish line. Unfortunately, the finish line came when the mouse stopped suddenly, but Jake did not.

It was a fairly gruesome crime scene, and while there was no little mouse-shaped chalk outline or yellow tape, the blood trail left little to be desired. The skidding of the front tire as it lost traction, the flattened mouse head sliding against the slick concrete— I'd say it was more like a blood smear.

Jake was iffy about having animals after that. He was afraid he'd accidentally kill them. Only five, it plagued his mind and caused him bad dreams. His internal monologue must have been frightening at that time and I'm glad I wasn't privy to it.

Then came a series of fish, all eventually flushed down the commode to join their brethren in the big koi pond in the sky.

Next, a succession of dogs and a cat, all unremarkable in that none died but a few had to be taken back to the pound when they didn't quite fit into our household. If they snapped at Jake once, all bets were off. They were evil and no amount of convincing in the world could remedy his fearful disdain.

The cat caused him a severe allergy attack, sending him to the hospital for a week with a collapsed lung. Yeah, that one left an impression on both of us. Nothing like a near-death experience to bring things into perspective.

Then there was the turtle he'd taken to play with outside, forgot, and returned to find shriveled like beef jerky inside its shell. It wasn't pretty, nor did it smell particularly appetizing.

But I believe the straw that broke the proverbial cliché, was him coming home to find the dried carcass of his *first* albino frog— Humbert Humbert is number two—glued to its climbing rock. That's what happens, I think, when you don't add enough water, put the bowl up on a shelf, forget about it for a week or so, and then take it down for inspection: *frog jerky*.

I'm pretty sure he expected to find his pet less … stale. It didn't help that the frog had died with its eyes and mouth open—as if screaming in agony in its final seconds of life.

Another coffee-induced memory included a sobbing seven-year-old entering the room with his shirt on inside out, and his shoes on the wrong feet.

"Mom, will I ever be normal?"

"Normal's overrated, honey. Why be normal when you can be different?" I always tried to play down the drama—temper his angst with flip one-liners, hoping he'd match my mood and bring down the urgency level. Jake's always at nine on a scale of one to ten—an emotional pot ready to boil over.

"Because different makes people look at me funny."

Screw other people, I wanted to say. Screw them and their neuro-typical brains. Screw anyone who can't live with a little diversity.

I think what I offered was a hug, and it served as a band-aid for a wound that would probably never heal: like wiping up a pool of blood with a single paper towel. Not nearly enough to do the job, even if you used the "quicker picker-upper."

Was I destined to be that albino frog? I felt much like it looked in death—my own inner howl threatening to break loose—a silent death wail. Or, was I that useless single-ply of toilet tissue, forever working hard to clean up messes that were way too big to handle? I felt forever not equal to the task and not even close to finding my inner bliss.

I stared at my husband, who was sitting on the couch across the room. He'd found some sort of comfort in the stagnant quo of our marriage—preferring to drown in a safe sea of reality TV programs and long naps—hunkered down and content to move through our life together from weekend to weekend, oblivious to the emotional rubble around us.

He was flipping through channels, clearly not expecting the next words out of my mouth.

"Yeah, I'm pretty sure I could get through the rest of my life if you never touched me again." I gripped my coffee cup, staring at the refrigerator, my eyes doing that thing they do when you've blurred out everything and can't quite focus.

"Excuse me?" My husband cut his eyes toward me, presumably thinking I was writing one of my screenplays and trying out a new line, aloud.

"Somewhere along the way, I've come to the conclusion that I'd be happier if you had a vagina, rather than a penis. And I mean this in the nicest possible way." A long sigh escaped my lungs—over-filled balloons thankfully shrinking back down to size.

"What the hell are you talking about?"

"I'm just saying, thanks for the use of your penis for the past twelve years, but I'm pretty sure I'm done. Think of it like a library book. It's overdue, but I'm bringing it back and now someone else can check it out."

It didn't come out exactly that way but you get the drift. Thing is, I hadn't expected him to say he loved me. Or that he wished I loved him in the same way. I hadn't expected to feel like such a shit. Especially since I'd pretty much given him *carte blanche* to go out and have sex with anyone he wanted as long as it wasn't me. It was an offhand remark, and I meant it, mostly out of guilt, but it would eventually come back to mock me.

At the time, I was Martin Luther King— I had a dream, and that dream didn't include raising two autistic kids on my own in a loveless marriage. But since I'd been pretty much doing that since they were born anyway, what was I holding on to? The scent of normalcy?

No, I think not. A whiff of desperation was more like it.

There was nothing normal about fielding questions about death from a five-year-old. Add to that Jaxson's newest obsession which involved stuffing multiple Hot Wheels cars down the commode. A severely strained septic system means a not-so-nice aroma hovering slightly under an oppressive cloud of Pine-Sol scent. Pine-Sol mixed with desperation is not the smell of a happy home.

My husband Will put down the remote. I had his complete attention. So I asked him to leave. He did, and my life pretty much went on as usual.

His absence lasted a week.

I called and asked him to come back when Jake approached me, seven days into our separation, and asked, "Mom, is this all a bad dream?"

Like the knife of guilt kids often wield, his wound was swift and slow to heal. I decided then and there that my personal happiness didn't make the top ten list. Because if *they* weren't happy (my kids), I wasn't happy anyway, so what was really the point? It wasn't like I was going out and looking for someone else. When you came with the kind of baggage where one made you check its ass for poop on a regular basis— and the other was prone to volcanic public displays—well, let's just say you ain't dating material. And, frankly, that was fine with me. My track record in that regard hadn't been stellar. Chock it up to severely impaired judgment—setting the bar a tad too low.

One only had to take a quick jog over to the way-back machine, jump in and set the dial back to the nineteen-eighties to get the general idea.

Like Scrooge and the Ghost of Christmas past . . .

1987: I lost my virginity at the age of seventeen to a basketball player five days before I graduated high school. He was a lovely, lovely boy and we were great friends, but at that point, all I really wanted to do was get it over with. My hymen was my stigmata and I wanted it gone.

It happened on the floor of my living room after school and basically I closed my eyes, held my breath, and waited for it all to be over.

Funny thing, but that's pretty much been my outlook on sex as a whole, ever since. Apathetic is what I'd probably call it. Sweet, sweet apathy— brand name Lexapro, in case you want some of your own.

My suspicion was that had I taken the vaginal route, rather than the penile one, things might have gone differently. I've never tested out my theory but I do hope to avail myself of the opportunity at some point. I know I'm physically attracted to both genders, but I'm fairly certain making a home with a female would have been a far more appropriate choice for me. I *like* women, generally speaking, more than men—and not in that fascist, male-bashing sort of way. I can simply relate to women more than men. I enjoy the company of women more than men.

And I'm trying to raise two of them, so that's a frightening concept.

I often think people were supposed to be sort of omni-sexual. Then something tragic happened along the way (*like fear mixed with ignorance: fignorance*), causing a split that would forever make it necessary to define ourselves, given our universal propensity for labeling things, to make the bitter pill we call life slightly easier to get down.

At any rate, what I do know is that the Whitman's Sampler of men I'd tried had led to the introduction of the antidepressant named above, so I was pretty sure I'd taken a wrong turn somewhere. Robert Frost's road less traveled might have been in order.

Instead, I married the first guy who asked.

I remember the night before my *first* wedding, asking one of my bridesmaids, "How do you know if you're in love?" It was eight hours before I'd be walking down the aisle in a ridiculously expensive dress with an equally ridiculous volume of satin material around my shoulder area.

I now know love is like the female orgasm. If you have to ask, you already know the answer. Because while *prior* to said orgasm things might feel all warm and tingly, you can't miss the actual thing any more than you can miss a sneeze or a fart.

Amy's answer hadn't been particularly helpful. "Um . . . I don't know. You just do. Is there something I need to know?"

I could have told her. She was a funny, great, engaging, brave girl and she'd have done it for me. She'd have taken one for the team and made it all go away. Calls would have been made, cigarettes would have been chain-smoked and I'd have been left to slink away quietly while she handled the shit storm. She thrived on that kind of stuff.

"No, I guess not." I wussed out. I would have never caused such a scandalous family ruckus. It just wasn't in my DNA. I wouldn't even send cold soup back at a restaurant. I didn't like to put people out. It was much easier to float downstream like a dead fish than to brave the cold waters like salmon do every year. Though, to be fair, salmon swim hundreds of miles against the tide, the sweet promise of spawning ahead, only to find death at the end of their pitiless trek. Presumably they don't see *that* coming.

Oh, Jesus! I was that *salmon*—in a designer white dress, and who the hell was I kidding with that color choice?

So I walked down the aisle, danced the first dance, drank some champagne, and cried myself to sleep on my wedding night.

Then, about a year and four months later, I divorced him. He was a nice guy, truly. I just woke up one day and thought, "I might have to take a dull Lady Bic to my wrist if I have to contemplate living here one more day." I felt like I couldn't breathe. The wrongness of the whole situation became palpable, but ended the night I told him I wanted a divorce.

"I'm sorry," I remember saying, a sloppy mess of tears and guilt.

"Don't be. I never thought you'd be brave enough to do it, but I knew it was coming," husband number one had confided.

Really? Because I had no clue he'd seen the writing on the wall. Today, this doesn't surprise me. How could I have been aware of how he was feeling if I wasn't even remotely self-aware?

And no sooner was I out of that relationship did I hop into another one, simply because I didn't want to be alone. I never considered the possibility that alone might be good. Quiet might be welcome. By the time I got pregnant, I knew my future was pretty much laid out, so why rage against the machine at that point?

What's done is done, I thought, with my seven-months-pregnant belly protruding toward the clerk of the court as my *second* husband and I exchanged vows at the back of a nothing-special room in the dilapidated courthouse downtown.

Then we went to Denny's and had breakfast. I think the entire day cost about forty bucks.

Then the whole autism thing snuck up on me like the swine flu— the symptoms fairly banal until it felt like I was hooked up to life support and a priest was administering last rites in the form of a cattle-prod shoved up my—

Okay, you get the drift . . .

After that, nothing else mattered. Will and I were raising a family, too busy making it from day to day unscathed to worry about such trifles as being in love. I knew it could be worse. I could be wearing a *burqa* and living in Afghanistan.

I came to the conclusion that there is no shame in playing the hand you are dealt.

There are, however, some rules.

—Try not to watch too many romantic comedies because they're fucking depressing and full of lies. That's not life. That's propaganda.

—Don't think of it as settling. Think of it as settling in for the long haul.

—Make the kids laugh at least once a day. It's a basic cure for all that ails you.

—And don't cry for me, Argentina. That'll just piss me off.

It took me a while, but I finally figured it out. In order to get where you want to be in life, sometimes you have to do stuff you don't want to do. In essence, and pardon the vulgar pun, but sometimes you have to suck a little cock. In art and commerce, in business and even in love (or lack thereof), there comes a moment when you have to decide: Am I a cock sucker or not?

To get things done, sometimes it's what's required— and if you're going to do something, for heaven's sake do it right. None of this namby-pamby spitting crap. If you're going to take the time to do it, take it to the head and swallow.

. . . then have a nice cuppa joe.

Making Movies of Myself

Jaxson is a little genius. I have no proof of this, but I think it might be true. He's a little guy for eight, and he packs a mean wallop when he wants to, but he is learning that tantrums won't get him what he wants. I've hauled him out of stores kicking and screaming on numerous occasions, bound and determined to come out the winner in our little Battle Royal.

He's finally getting it. Thus his aggression is getting much better.

Here are a few tidbits about him of interest:

He grinds his teeth— a sound that sets my own incisors on edge. I'm pretty sure I've developed a Tourette's-like eye tic because of it.

He likes to have three televisions in the house on at all times, each with volumes raised to an ear-splitting decibel level. I've learned to tune them out and move through the white noise with general ease, though on some days even Calgon couldn't take me far enough away.

He doesn't like being clothed. Every day he gets off the school van, hops inside, and proceeds to remove everything he's wearing except his undies. Rain or shine, summer or winter—Jaxson doesn't like being dressed.

He attends a regular elementary school and even participates in a general education first grade classroom throughout the day when he's not in his learning disabled class with his other special *compadres*.

If he were left alone in the house, if for some reason the rest of us suddenly disappeared from his world, I have no doubt he'd make it until either the food ran out or he set the house on fire—whichever came first.

And around here, we know a little bit about fire. The one time since his birth I dozed off while reading, Jaxson set his bedroom on fire. With a lighter I'd accidentally left in an old purse, deep in the back of my closet. Now, every lighter, knife, box, bottle or jar of medication, and every Sharpee marker I own, are on permanent lockdown. The key is hidden and moved randomly, just in case the little bugger decides to play Hercule Poirot.

Jaxson can make his own popcorn in the microwave, toast his own waffles, cook his own chicken nuggets, and apply a liberal amount of catsup to the plate for dipping.

He also has an affinity for baths, of which he takes at least two a day, filming his watery antics for posterity. Filmmaking is his newest obsession and no less than fourteen digital video cameras have paid for it with their lives. One after the other have met their demise as Jaxson runs around the house capturing his tomfoolery digitally before he plays it back for his own amusement, eventually putting the camera in the toilet or under the running tap.

One day he discovered the USB port and plugged a camera into my PC, immediately figuring out how to upload the footage. He was seven and only slightly verbal at the time. When he somehow found out how to pull the footage into my video editing software and create a DVD, I began to have concerns.

The advent of digital media has been a great technological accomplishment, but with it comes certain problems. My child doesn't understand that it might not be interesting or even particularly appropriate for someone to video themselves taking a bowel movement and then play it over and over on the big screen television in the living room during Thanksgiving Dinner. While *I* can fully appreciate how he adjusted the camera for maximum viewing benefit, getting the lighting just so, panning in for a close-up, others may not concur.

Needless to say, he's not getting my AOL password.

I saw what happened to that couple who took innocent pictures of their three kids in the tub and brought them to their local megastore to be developed. Next thing they knew, they were handcuffed as Child Protective Services carted off their kids for a month's stay in foster care. Video evidence of my child taking a poop—his little Vienna sausage dangling in the frame—posted to the Boob Tube would cause a considerably greater stir.

I assume the benefits of lockdown would include three squares a day cooked by someone other than me, and all the time to sleep I required. But that fantasy would probably be forgotten about the time they implemented the full body cavity search. And I have no desire to be deloused.

The great thing is, Jaxson actually caught his first poop in the toilet on camera. The long wait as his plaintive stare took up the entire video screen, camera sitting on the edge of the bathroom sink. The look of revelation in his widened eyes as he peeked from the camera to the contents of the bowl beneath him, then back to the camera, his brow furrowed, wondering if what he'd just done was something he'd want to repeat again. Him wiping himself with a look of disgust before tossing the soiled toilet paper and standing to pull up his undies before flushing.

"Gotcha!" he'd proudly exclaimed as the turd disappeared into oblivion.

And then he washed his hands! Oh, glorious day—it's right there on film. HE WASHED HIS HANDS!

People look for miracles everywhere these days, trying to make something of nothing— the Virgin Mary from a smear of mustard on a hamburger bun, the sweat stain on Uncle Joe's work shirt that looks suspiciously like Elvis.

To me, *these* little moments are my miracles.

He pooped in the toilet!

He threw his soiled undies in the hamper by himself!

By summer he'd amassed so much video footage, I compiled a folder on my hard drive and began pulling the clips up one by one, putting a movie together for the family.

Merry Christmas! Jaxson Makes a Movie!

During the course of this, I found some footage that was a bit disturbing, considering these were things I hadn't even known happened. He's never out of my sight for long but often when he's playing outside, I'm sitting on the lawn with a book in my lap and I guess I missed a few things. Like the footage of his little fingers as he pulled a red berry from a tree, popping it into his mouth.

It's great that he had the presence of mind to then turn the camera on his face as he chewed— the pucker on his lips providing evidence it wasn't exactly tasty. But after he popped the next four in his mouth in succession, I became concerned. We had always called these Choke Berries. I looked at the date on the footage, realizing it had been taken three days earlier. Well, he hadn't choked, so crisis averted.

Then there was the fifteen-minute clip of him crying. That day he hadn't been in trouble, so I could only assume he'd needed a good cry— he had this drama queen energy going and was just wailing for the camera as he sat in his room alone. Tears streamed down his face as he set the camera on his Little Tykes desk and threw his hands up in the air, as if pondering the weight of the world on his tiny shoulders.

Shaking his head, he buried his face in his hands and his howling took on a fevered pitch. I felt so sad as I watched, wondering what the poor child was so upset about. Where had I gone wrong?

Then he abruptly stopped crying, pulled his face up to look at the camera and smiled.

The little *shit*! He was acting! And doing a pretty damned good job of it, too.

The Academy Award goes to . . .

His speech was also improving. He began to pick up little phrases here and there and often parroted them back at appropriate times, telling me his brain was starting to make some meaningful connections.

If Mommy began to yell when he started tossing drinking glasses on the kitchen floor to see what they looked like as they shattered, he'd say, "you okay?" This is what I ask him when he's upset or has hurt himself and he repeats it back to me in the same rhythm and tone as I say it. "You okay?" "It's okay . . ."

But if I reply, "No, it's not okay. Now Mommy has to sweep glass up off the floor, and I'm pretty sure she's on the verge of a cranial bleed. So, it's definitely not okay!" He will continue his verbal assault, "U okay? It's okay . . . " until I agree with him that it is okay. He even patted me on the head once consolingly, as I wilted under the pressure.

He's just not getting that it's his behavior which causes my anguish. He sees that I've dissolved into a puddle of muffled sobs but is unable to take the thought process one step further: *Oh, she's upset because I took the entire box of glass Christmas ornaments from the basement and broke them all over my brothers' bedroom floor.*

That was another disturbing clip I found out about after it occurred, because I'd committed the unmitigated crime of taking a shower.

Lately he's begun singing the theme songs from sitcoms and commercials, as well as memorizing odd phrases from whatever he happens to be watching or listening to at the time.

Needless to say, I try to avoid *South Park* until he's fast asleep. Third grade cartoon boys cursing a blue streak on TV = good. First grade human boys doing same in class = not so much.

"Any ninnit. Wafer it. Wafer it." (Translation: Any minute. Wait for it. Wait for it.) "Ah . . . Good job!"

Usually I don't know the context of the phrase he's repeating. I'm left wondering: did he hear me say this, or was it Curious George? Or was he wandering the house at midnight as we all slumbered, somehow tuning in to a documentary on cable?

I'm a heavy sleeper, so the latter is a definite possibility.

Somewhere he picked up the little nugget, "Boo-ya!"

Okay, so "Boo-ya" works if, say, he's managed to putt his little plastic ball into the mouth of his alligator golf game.

But "Boo-ya" is decidedly less amusing when he says it after kicking me in the shin.

"Boo-ya this, little man," I say, grabbing my right butt cheek and leaning in for a kiss.

Of course, he repeats exactly what Mommy does.

"Boo-ya this!" he mimics, grabbing his butt and smiling.

Yeah, that one should go over real well at school.

Juggling Act

As winter approaches and the leaves fall from the trees, I get this impending sense of doom: an isolation brought on by lots of snow and too much time spent inside.

I also tend to live too far in my head—thinking too much, wanting too much, dreaming too much.

Driving alone always makes me feel better. I'm rarely by myself, so it's a cherished novelty. Nobody needing me, wanting me for something or encroaching on my sense of self. In the car, I turn up the radio full blast and sing my ass off.

While I'm certain hearing a recording of my vocal talents would make me cringe, in the moment I'm a star, entertaining the world with my obviously untapped musical brilliance.

On this particular day, I was headed for a conference with Jake's teacher— nothing amiss, just the quarterly check-in to make sure we were all on the same page.

I'm not sure what set me off. It could have been attributed to my period, or the depressing sight of all of the fog and naked trees devoid of color, or the two loads of laundry waiting to be folded when I returned home.

Had any tractors or farm vehicles passed me on the empty country road, they'd have been treated to quite a show. As the radio blared, I started bawling. With my car flying past horses and cow pastures, I had myself a good cry to the lyrics of Traffic's *Feelin' All Right*.

"Ya' feelin' allright? Wo-hoo. Not feelin' too good myself . . . "
Sob, sob, sob.
Gooey, snotty nose— wiped on the back of my sleeve.
"Ya' feelin' allright? I'm not feelin' too good myself . . . "
Sob, cough, sob some more.

There was absolutely no impetus for my sudden case of waterworks. Neither of the children had done anything upsetting that morning. The day was going quite well, actually. I was in my favorite place: alone in the car, speeding down the quiet countryside.

As I pulled into the school parking lot, I got my act together, wiped my face and headed inside, wondering if getting off that antidepressant, years earlier, had been a wise decision. Apathy was preferable to sudden bouts of hysterical sobbing. Who needs to feel anything when you can go through life as numb as Joan Rivers' lips?

I spent the next two hours sharing funny stories about Jake with his teachers, who added to my future writing fodder by sharing some precious moments I'd otherwise not be privy to.

"We let the kids keep water bottles in class and they can fill them up from the water fountains. Anyway, Jake asked if he could go fill his up and I said sure," his teacher said, elaborating on one of many stories I heard that day. "So, he hadn't come back, and I wondered what had happened. I see Jake clutching his water bottle and moaning next to the water fountain. I say, 'Jake, what's up, buddy?' and he's moaning . . ." Here, she starts laughing. "It took a few minutes for me to understand him. He's clutching his water bottle and drinking out of it, but every time he takes a sip, he's gagging. So I say, 'What's wrong, Jake?' And he points and says, really loud: 'Someone vomited in the water fountain. What's wrong with people?'"

I'm already giggling because I can picture it with perfect clarity— kids passing him in the hall, rubbernecking their way back to class as his teacher tried to bring him down.

What my son hasn't seemed to put together yet is that his outbursts and odd activities in public only single him out even further from his peers. A friend very adeptly likened his mind to a road map where many of the streets had been erased. He was unable to get from point A to point B because the connection between two points simply didn't exist and the rerouting took too long.

"So I get to the fountain, and teachers are popping their heads out of rooms, and I look into the water fountain and, sure enough, it looked like someone had spit in the water fountain, little food particles or something . . . Not a lot, mind you. Just enough to send him over the edge."

"Oh, God!" I clamp a hand over my mouth, trying not to laugh any louder than I already am.

"Oh, yeah. He freaked out. But, what I didn't get was that he kept sipping from the water bottle, gagging, and then holding it out in front of him, toward me. He finally gasped and said, 'I just know some puke got into my water bottle.'"

"I'm like, Jake *stop* drinking from it for a minute. It was as if he was locked in a tic or something. He was grossed out, but couldn't stop sipping from the bottle. Sipping and gagging, sipping and gagging. And staring at the wad of spit."

I let out a snort of laughter. I could see Jake bent over the water fountain, riveted to the glob of whatever but unable to look away, dry heaving after each sip.

"I tried to explain to him that there's no way the spit or vomit or whatever it was made it into his bottle. I even showed him how, when he filled the bottle from the fountain, the water never touched the bottom but went right into his bottle."

"Oh, dear God," I said, wiping tears from my eyes.

"Anyway, that's why I sent the note home on Friday for you to send in a new water bottle for him. When I finally pried the other one out of his clammy hands, I tossed it in the trash. Problem solved."

"You guys sure don't get paid enough." I sighed, and started to go through Jake's "bad feelings" folder. It was clear by the scrawl on the pages which days had been worse for him. On some, the writing was legible and neatly confined to the lines on the paper. On others, the words trailed downward, spiraling out of control, mirroring his emotions.

10-29-09

I am not feeling right today. I don't like it that my Mom likes other boys liping. It's gross. I don't like it that she likes cemeteries either.

"What's this one about?" his teacher asked, tapping her pencil eraser on the page in front of me.

"Liping? What's lip—"

Oh, shit. I remember that morning. The discussion about gay boys. Liping was kissing, I presumed.

Oops . . .

Well, to be fair, *he* had broached the subject and I'd only briefly explained homosexuality. I can only surmise that while I was giving him a very banal, very PC version of two boys who liked one another, what he was visualizing was some lip on lip action. My explanation was about feelings—his interpretation followed through to the physical aspect.

"Kissing," I cleared it up for them. "We were talking about two boys kissing."

"Ah," the teacher said, biting her lip. "That explains that one. What about the cemeteries?"

Okay, so that one was an error in judgment. On the same morning of the "liping" discussion, we'd been running a bit early on our way to school. I won't leave him there too early because I don't like the idea of him standing alone outside for too long, subject to a large group of waiting kids surrounding him.

That is a formula for disaster.

Any number of things could happen to mar any possibility of him having a decent day. Little did I know at the time, I'd managed to decimate his mood that day all on my own.

I explained to his teacher that to eat up some time I'd taken a short ride through the cemetery a block from the school. I happen to like cemeteries. I find them quite peaceful—lovely in fact. Jake hadn't expressed any concern at the time—we'd even rolled down the windows and marveled at the very old dates on some of the headstones.

It's not like we got out and traipsed over sacred ground or embarked upon some weird blood-letting ritual. We'd taken a little drive down the tiny, curving road that led from one end of the cemetery to the other. No big deal.

I'd thought wrong.

"So what happened when he got here?" I asked, only now realizing I'd started off his day with a little tiptoe around death. It never occurred to me this would be disturbing to him.

"He asked us if we liked cemeteries. I said I did, and Linda said she didn't. He didn't make a big deal about it, but he wrote this down in his feelings folder. And he was a bit of a mess the rest of the day."

NOTE TO SELF: Steer clear of cemeteries in future.

"Well, I won't do *that* again," I promised.

"We'd appreciate it," the paraprofessional said with a giggle. God bless her.

How could I have not seen that would be an issue? Am I so far from being the average parent that I couldn't put two and two together and realize that driving through a place where dead people reside for all eternity wasn't a prudent choice?

I might as well have said, "We all die at some point, Jake, but hey, look at the pretty flowers people will leave for you. Oh, and have a nice day, honey."

They shared a few more stories of teachers who had begun working with Jake on a one-on-one basis. Like the computer teacher Jake liked because of his handlebar moustache. He often came to the rescue when he saw Jake being bothered by other kids in the halls.

At the beginning of the year, as we'd passed through the computer room for orientation, Jake had approached the computer teacher, looked straight at him and said, "How do you make your moustache do that?"

Jake wasn't interested in checking out the computers, didn't have any questions about the new school, he only wanted to find out about the cool facial hair. To his credit, the computer teacher spent a few minutes explaining the ins and outs of moustache wax.

The gym teacher had also made an impression, shooting baskets with Jake when he noticed him feeling isolated and insecure within his peer group.

"You're pretty good at this, Jake," coach had told him after spending their fifteen minutes of free time shooting hoops with him, one on one.

His teacher told me Jake beamed with delight and felt special for the rest of the day. This is something new for him—these adult male advocates taking time around others to encourage something he's interested in.

I was never able to attribute my ridiculous crying jag from earlier in the day to anything specific, but during the drive home, I got choked up again. This time I knew the reason.

I thought about the great educators my children have the privilege of being mentored by. My life definitely fits into the "it takes a village to raise a child" category. I couldn't pull this off on my own and I'm glad I don't have to because sometimes it feels like my life is one big juggling act.

Thank heaven for the people out there who catch the ball when I drop it because I have a lot of balls in the air on any given day and I'm bound to drop a few along the way.

"The . . ."
(a free association exercise)
by Jake Lopez

The chair you sit on
The light you light
The games you play
The things you learn
The school everyone hates
The tuning fork you use
The marker you use
The camera you take pictures with
The little things
The big things
The square things
The round things
The things you eat
The plants you grow
The notebook you draw in
The time you do something
The magnifying glass you use
The computers you play
The things you think
The people around you
The thing you do
The color that you like
The place you live
The things you want
They are all the things.

Jehovah's at My Door

Her name was Sue and she found the time to visit me once a week, each Tuesday.

The first time I opened the door, using my leg to block three-year-old Jaxson from escaping through the crack, she smiled and held up a copy of *The Watchtower*.

"Hi. I'm Sue. How would you like to strengthen your relationship with the Lord? All it takes is fifteen minutes a day!"

I'm pretty sure the Lord would need a bit more of my time. You know, for lengthy explanations of my transgressions and a detailed list of how I might do better in the future.

I was raised a Catholic and taught there was no fast track to heaven. Lots of praying, confession, and wallowing in guilt were necessary in order to be in the Big Guy's good graces.

The sisters at Saint Charles Catholic School were quite the sadistic, habit-wearing bunch. I recall Sister Ethel telling us that babies who weren't baptized went to purgatory and it was our duty to pray for them nightly. Each of our prayers would set one tiny soul free, and as a good boy or girl, it was our duty to save them.

I often wondered if Sister Ethel ever stopped to think about the repercussions of sharing this tidbit of Catholic information with our malleable young minds.

I, for one, stayed up late into the night saying my Hail Marys and Our Fathers, counting how many babies I'd saved and trying not to fall asleep before I beat the number of the previous night. None of those babies were going to hell on my watch and my final grade in Algebra probably spoke to the lack of sleep I got.

At any rate, this fifteen-minute thing Jehovah's handmaiden was offering sounded kind of appealing—though I admit I briefly thought of those weight-eliminating machines the infomercials hawked on late night television promising fast results for only ten monthly installments of nineteen ninety-five.

Burn me once, shame on me. Burn me twice . . .

Sue continued her weekly visits, much to my chagrin, mostly because I never did enough to discourage her. But the day she handed me a copy of *The Watchtower* with a sketch of a slouching young man on the cover—hands hiding his face—I had a moment.

The headline on the front page read: WHAT DOES GOD THINK OF THE HOMOSEXUAL?

Let's just say, this one got me feeling a little . . . irritated.

I stared at the headline as she opened her Bible, readying herself for the weekly verse she shared with me.

"How *does* Jehovah feel about same-sex marriage?"

The corners of Sue's mouth dipped slightly.

This was a test. Of course I knew how the rest of this conversation would go but I felt the need to have her elaborate.

"Well, God intended marriage to be between a man and woman. Homosexuality is a sin . . . "

Oh man. She's gonna make me do it.

As a young girl when someone said or did something I disagreed with, I just let it slide. The kid bullying the smaller guy on the playground, the adult saying the "n" word— I'd just cringe and look the other way.

But as an adult, I feel . . . *ugly* if I do that.

Because when I was twelve and riding my bike in flip-flops and Rodney Lloyd, the cute guy from down the block, came to my rescue when I ran over a rock and slid to a stop, causing more than a bit of damage to the skin of my toes.

I was the "average" girl. Boys didn't usually come riding to my aid, probably because they didn't need to be associating with someone they didn't want to feel up.

But Rodney scooped me up and carried me home, wiping the gravel off my feet after setting me down in my yard.

But the *why* was what got me—the why of his actions. We were buddies and Rodney was that elusive teenager who didn't feel the need to make others feel like pond scum.

Rodney was the man!

I decided I'd pay it forward. It took me a few years to muster the courage but eventually I did. And once I started, there was no stopping me.

I wouldn't let things go when I felt something needed to be said.

"The good news is," Sue continued, "God can help homosexuals overcome their aberrant attractions and tendencies so that they can gain His blessings. We are very tolerant of those who wish to abstain from certain behaviors and overcome their same-sex attractions."

"Uh huh . . . " I paused to grab a cigarette, lighting it in silence for effect.

I presumed smoking was another no-no, but barring my ability to do something more shocking in her presence, I opted for a stogie. I needed a moment to gather my thoughts.

"So, that's a no on the same-sex marriage thing?" I really was going for discomfort: hers.

"Well, yes." She smiled again, but I could see it in her eyes. She knew she had lost me.

"You know . . . it occurs to me that using the word tolerance doesn't generally work when you're happy to stop by and try to recruit someone of homosexual affiliation, though admit that if they aren't willing to 'abstain from certain behaviors' they won't be getting into the Kingdom of Heaven. Forgive me, but that's slightly offensive.

"Well, I certainly don't mean to be offensive—"

"—of course not." My smile matched hers. "Nobody ever *means* to be offensive."

Our time together was coming to an end—we both knew it as we said our goodbyes that day and I closed the door.

"Ca-Ca," Jaxson said as he flew through the living room on his Big Wheel, tires getting very little traction against the slick wood floor.

"You got that right, buster," I said, quickly moving out of his way, "That was a bunch of ca-ca."

To her credit, she came back one more time. Jehovah would have been proud of her tenacity.

But on the next Tuesday, I was ready.

As I opened the door to her for the last time, her smile disappeared as she stared down at my new t-shirt.

I'd found a great sketch of two boys kissing on the Internet, printed out the iron-on transfer and then applied it to a hot pink t-shirt.

Because I've been blessed with more than my share of boobage, the picture stretched pornographically across my chest, and her eyes were riveted to the hot zone.

I didn't get a Bible verse that day, just another sad little pamphlet that I tossed into the recycle bin with the rest of them—all on their way to becoming part of something else.

Something . . . useful.

Shame on Me

"Mom, did I get any letters yet?" Jake hovered behind me as I sat at my computer, checking my emails and having my morning coffee.

"No, honey."

"Did you check the mail?"

"Yes I did."

"Your email?"

"Uh huh, nothing yet."

It had been five months and Jake hadn't heard back from the Big Yellow Video Game Character whose name was no longer in my vocabulary. Jake asked daily—not once daily, but multiple times a day—much to the exasperation of my irritable bowel.

But it wasn't the Obnoxious Yellow Gibberish-Speaking Entity from Hell that chapped my ass that day. As it turned out, more pressing issues arose.

My first mistake of the day had been the assumption that I could take a nice relaxing bubble bath without interference.

I'd poured a generous amount of rose petal bubble bath into the tub and waited for it to fill. The bottle promised it was "gently infused with rose crystals, accented by geranium essence . . . unabashedly feminine."

I slipped into the girly-water, soaking for what seemed like a heavenly eternity when Jax flew into the room with his father's cell phone to his ear.

Yeah, that was a no-no for a plethora of reasons, including but not limited to the fact he'd once racked up fifty dollars worth of charges when he found actual pay-per-play games on the cell just the push of a button away.

Clearly many buttons had been pushed.

"Gimme that, you," I reached for the phone but he backed up and giggled.

"Uh huh," he pretended to carry on a conversation, "what you say?"

"Give it, mister." I stretched as far as possible, sending geranium and rose-scented bubbles across the carpet as he stayed just out of reach.

"Wassa matter?" he asked his pretend friend—God, I hoped it was a pretend friend and not someone in China or Yemen. Those ten-cents-a-minute minutes were ticking away . . .

"Jaxson. Give it to me *now*." He tossed it to me and ran. Thankfully I caught it before it hit the rose-scented water. Checking the display, I said a little *gracias* to the man upstairs after realizing no call had actually been made.

My second mistake of the day was checking the outgoing call log. Just for giggles.

That, I probably shouldn't have done, because curiosity doesn't always kill the cat. Curiosity sometimes just pisses the cat off. A pissed off cat is much more dangerous than a dead one. And, at present, I was one pissed off pussy.

Jake peeked his head into the bathroom, covering his eyes with his hands. "Mom, when you get out are you going to check your email again?"

"Jake, honey. Please. I'm begging you." I snapped the phone closed, the reality of what I'd just learned sinking in. I don't think I have to spell it out. Let's just say there was a name and number in that cell phone that didn't belong in that cell phone.

For all intents and purposes, Will and I live a marriage of convenience— roommates with occasional benefits—though *I'd* personally be loathe to describe them as benefits, I'm pretty sure he does. Okay, I'm guessing on that one because this isn't something we discuss. Following the week of separation years earlier, we both just dug in our heels and kept busy with the day-to-day stuff— stuck on a sinking ship, too busy tossing water overboard to stop and discuss the weather. We'd settled into a comfortable life whereby I take care of the kids and the house, he brings home a paycheck, and neither of us asks too many questions. We're kind and respectful to one another, but nobody is going to be mistaking us for John and Yoko.

Still, I assumed since *I* wasn't partaking of any extra-curricular shenanigans—

"Mom?" Jake whined, jarring me back to reality.

"I'll check later, I promise. Now let Mommy finish her bath, okay?"

"Okay, Mom. I love you."

"I love you too, buddy."

I lay back in the water, submerging myself while pondering my next move.

Two hours later, I was at the grocery store, having left both kids with their father after mentioning to him that the tub was in dire need of attention. The grout needed scrubbing.

Did he, perhaps, have a cleaning product he could recommend? Oh, and I also handed him his cell phone and smiled.

A nice, big, *I-know-what-you-did* smile—just so we were on the same page.

After returning home from the store, unpacking the bags, and heading to the bathroom to put the toiletries away, I knew.

My suspicions that he'd done something naughty were confirmed when I saw the sparkling white bathroom before me. The sink was immaculate, I noticed, as I put the new shampoo, soap, and toothpaste under the counter.

Someone had been guilt-cleaning.

I knew I had no right to be upset. He'd gone out and done exactly what I'd suggested he do years earlier—even if what I suggested had been an off-hand remark meant to assuage my own guilt more than anything else. Because, I'm guessing, once your wife puts the crystal clear image of her preference for vagina over penis into your mind, it's kind of hard for the average Joe to forget. Still, we'd never agreed on anything, and I just assumed he'd continue to do what I was doing— shove my own wants and needs aside and concentrate on the kids.

Suddenly, without any ground rules, we were in uncharted, turbulent waters.

Go ahead. Go out—be fruitful, just don't multiply because that's a head-ache I don't need right now.

I'd been so distracted by the clean bathroom, I didn't immediately notice Jaxson at the bottom of the now mold-free tub, lying on his stomach, humping the almost empty bathtub with wild abandon. That's something he's done regularly since about the age of eighteen months. The kid will dry hump anything that doesn't move. The living room floor, his bed, my bed, his brother's bed or floor . . . the list is endless.

Rose-scented bubbles covered his little body as he held his head up over the white foam. The carpet beneath my feet, I now noticed, was sopping wet and an "unabashedly feminine" scent squished out from between my toes. It seemed someone had found my bubble bath.

"Hey there, buddy. Having fun?" I smiled, but my heart wasn't in it.

All I could think about was the unabashed, moldy dry rot that would linger long after the scent of rose had gone. Well, that and how my amateur sleuthing had forced my husband into scrubbing his shame away.

Guilt. That is what I felt and, frankly, it left me a little . . . perturbed.

Why should I feel guilty? It's not out of the realm of reasoning that a man could and should clean a bathroom now and again.

But heading back into the kitchen to see the man of the house taking a scouring pad and Ajax to the dirty stove sent me over the edge.

"Mom, don't forget my letters," Jake yelled from his room.

I came to a dead stop in the center of the living room.

Scrub, scrub, scrub . . .

"Did you hear me, Mom?"

I sat down to my computer and logged on with a silence that must have read like impending doom.

Beep. You've Got Mail.

Sigh. Yeah, I always have mail. What emissary from Calcutta needs my help disbursing his vast wealth this week?

Scrub, scrub, scrub—then the clatter of iron stove burners being removed.

A slight facial tic and that impending sense of doom again.

"Did I get anything, Mom?"

Oh, *Jesus wept*!

Let me just say, I am not proud of what happened next. It was highly uncalled for. I'd blame it on my period but it was nowhere near that time of month.

I'd blame it on the guy in the kitchen scrubbing away the shame, but he hadn't done anything I hadn't pushed him into.

I take full responsibility. I am not proud. I am a very bad person.

Scrub, scrub, clatter.

"Mom, did I *get any letters?*"

"*No Jake, you did not get any letters! They did not send them on a train! They did not ship them on a plane! They have not come by cab or canoe! There is no fucking mail for you!*"

"Mom!"

"Jen!" Anger from the man presently wearing yellow gloves and holding a dripping scouring pad.

I don't like anger.

I *feel* it—I just make an effort not to express it. It's rarely helpful.

"I'm sorry, Jake." *Shame on me.*

"Why are you mad?" Jake stood just behind his bedroom door.

"I'm not mad, buddy. I'm tired. We'll check again tomorrow, okay?"

"Okay Mom. I love you."

"I love you too, buddy."

Poor kid. All he wanted was to know if a letter from Pokemon had arrived and I lambaste him with a highly inappropriate Seussical reference.

He disappeared into his room just as Jaxson turned up the volume on the television because my little outburst had infringed on his ability to repeatedly replay a fifteen-second clip of *Blue's Clues* and hear it without interruption.

Scrub, scrub, scrub. The man in the kitchen continued his guilt-cleaning in silence.

Jealous.

I had to look it up to make sure of what I was feeling, and since I was already sitting at the computer, I did just that.

Jealous, adj.

1. Envious: feeling bitter and unhappy because of another's advantages, possessions or luck.
2. Suspicious of rivals: feeling suspicious about a rival's or competitor's influence, especially in regard to a loved one

3. Watchful: possessively watchful of something
4. Demanding loyalty: demanding exclusive loyalty or adherence

As I pondered the definition, it was clear I didn't fall into category number two. I honestly didn't care what he did. Have at it, baby. Your body's a wonderland. I just don't want to hear about it. I don't want it in my face so that I know you're out there tripping the frigging light fantastic while I snake the toilet drain for the fifth time this week.

Yesterday, I found a tube of toothpaste in there, for God's sake!

NOTE TO SELF: Replace *his* tube with the one presently at the bottom of the bathroom trash can— yeah, the one that'd previously spent a little quality time in the bowels of the toilet drain.

Take that!

Number four worked for me though I wasn't proud of the fact. But why should he be dialing inappropriate numbers and doing God Knows What while I snake toilet drains?

Where's my fucking bliss?

Bitter, party of one, your table is ready.

I could probably use some of that apathy right about now because, frankly, I want to get out there and feel something for a minute or two that doesn't involve unsent letters from the Rudest Yellow Cartoon Video Game Character In The Free World, daily ass checks for poo, and Humpy Humperson over there who was, by the way, busy dry humping a towel in the middle of the living room floor.

C'est la vie.

Today, *ma vie* sucketh the big one.

But tomorrow is another day.

. . . and tomorrow, and tomorrow, and tomorrow.

The old cliché about making our own beds then having to lie in them might be overused, but in this case it's my truth. So, my bed is full of crumbs. So what? It's still a bed—a place to rest my head at the end of the day. The crumbs don't negate the bed: they just make sleeping a bit less comfortable.

Shit

Poop has played a larger role in my life than I'd like.

Both my kids have had toileting issues—Jake refuses to wipe with anything but baby wipes and he has no problem asking me to check his rear to establish its cleanliness.

It is a real conundrum.

I can be in the bathroom and hear him hovering just outside, "Mom, are you going pee or poo?"

Now, here's the thing—I learned pretty darned quickly he needed to believe that Mom doesn't poo. Urine can flow as freely as Niagara Falls, but I'd made the mistake of answering truthfully with regard to the body excretion most foul once, and he lost his . . . *shit.*

"Mom! Oh, yuck! Don't go poo while I'm at home!" I heard his bedroom door slam across the house.

There may be a lot I'm willing to do for my kids, but holding it in isn't one of them.

People need to evacuate. It's just natural.

But, God forbid, when anything even remotely related to the topic of number two comes up while he's eating, he'll just open his mouth and the food will fall where it lands.

His dish will be emptied of whatever is on it, then tossed into the sink, and the last thing you'll hear are his feet stomping across the floor, "God, I hate this house!"

In the pooping department, we, his family, are the enemy and not to be trusted.

When he was in kindergarten, I got a call from the school nurse. Jake wouldn't poop at school, ever, but one day an emergent situation arose, thereby necessitating release. Noticing his discomfort, his teacher sent him to the nurse who asked enough questions to ascertain the problem. She then provided a quiet single bathroom in her office, promised to leave the room, and let him do his business in peace.

I learned all this when the chuckling vice-principal gave me a call at home. Jake was fairly notorious within the small school already, such were his eccentric behaviors in class. Just the week previous, he'd told his paraprofessional that she had bad breath and could she please not talk to him.

Looking back, it would have been really nice if they'd added up repeatedly running out of the classroom, toileting issues, sensory issues, and inept socialization, and come up with autism. But that's not how it ended up playing out.

"Okay, Mrs. Lopez, what's up with the bathroom situation? Is this new?"

If only.

"Um, nope. He said he never pooped at school."

"Well today he didn't have much choice. It's fine, I don't mind letting him go in here when he needs it, but can you tell me a little bit about the mirror?"

"Mirror? What mirror?" At the time this was new, even to me.

"He requested a mirror so he could check himself." I could picture it—I was probably on speaker phone and the entire office staff were shoving their morning donuts down their gullets and listening in.

While she found this amusing, I did not. This was my baby. He was a tiny little kindergartner and it had taken an entire week for him to stop crying in class all day. Literally, from the time I dropped him off to the time I picked him up in the afternoon, he'd cried. To say it was traumatic for us both would be an understatement.

On most days, I'd just stare at the clock, paralyzed with anxiety, praying for it to hit three o'clock so I could rush over and pick him up.

I pondered home schooling, though I laugh at the thought now. Home schooling? Please. I can't get him to shit properly and I think I can teach him to read and learn his multiplication tables?

I'll leave the teaching to the professionals.

I could hear her shuffling papers on her desk. "I don't know what he's checking. I assumed you'd know. Should I go in there and—"

"No! Do *not* open the door and interrupt him!"

God, that would scar him for life. He'd never feel safe in any bathroom, ever, and I didn't need him crapping into plastic bags in his bedroom closet.

"I'll give him a few more minutes. He was so cute— he asked if I had a mirror and some baby wipes and the poor kid looked like he was about to burst. So I went out to my car and got my little compact makeup mirror and luckily I had some wet ones in there too."

Suddenly it came to me, "Oh, he's checking to see if he's wiped himself clean."

"Ahhh," came the chorus of now clued-in voices, substantiating my earlier guess about the speaker phone.

Ok, party's over, people. Nothing more to see here. Move along.

Then, years later, came the pigs and their shit.

We moved from Florida to Michigan, where we now live on a farm. My mom and stepdad, Bob, bought a house on fifty acres of magnificent fields and woods, and we built a home on the property they were more than willing to share.

The first year Bob bought eight pigs and the boy who formerly washed his hands fifty times a day, instantly became The Pig Whisperer.

Jake, tentative at first, eventually got into the pen with them, sat on the ground and was able to feed them by hand.

This I just couldn't understand.

He hated discussing poop, he was obsessed with antibacterial hand wash, but he could sit in a pig pen where the smell was so bad, I could barely tolerate it. If he understood they were basically wallowing in their own effluent, it didn't seem to register.

I saw trouble brewing when he started naming the pigs— where he saw pets, the rest of us saw pork chops. Lots and lots of "the other white meat" would eventually be shrink-wrapped and fill the freezers in the barn. But before that would happen, we'd fatten them up with pig feed and food scraps we'd normally trash, that now went into slop buckets.

Jake visited his new friends daily, giving each steadily growing piggy a moniker, most of which elude me now. Except for Petunia, Sad Eyes, Mr. P. and Jake's favorite, Daisy.

I, like most adults who eat meat, try not to personalize something we're eventually going to ingest. Normally I prefer picking my meat up at the grocery store where it bears no resemblance to the animal it once was. I find it aids in the digestion of said meat.

When we got the pigs, my mom and I sat Jake down and had a little discussion regarding the food chain and the circle of life. Humans, we told him, often like to eat meat. Humans who want to eat meat not tainted by preservatives, steroids and antibiotics, raise the meat themselves. Meat comes from animals. That bacon he enjoys, I told him, once looked like his new friends.

We wanted to make sure he understood that at the end of the day, Daisy, Sweet Eyes, Petunia, Mr. P, and the rest of their porcine pals would end up on the dinner table.

It's hard to say what he was actually thinking at the time because he seemed okay with what was going to eventually happen. The only thing he made us promise was that Daisy go to one of the other family members to eat. Not him, by God— he was not interested in eating her.

Driving Miss Daisy, sure. Riding Miss Daisy, absolutely. Rolling around in her crap, *no problemo*.

Eating her— not a chance in hell.

By the end of the summer the pigs were so huge they were frightening to look at. When they started escaping the pen, other issues arose. Pig wrangling, while funny to the outside observer, isn't quite so funny when one of them is snorting and chasing you around the yard.

My first clue that something was amiss came when Jaxson ran into the living room pulling on his clothes and pointing out the window yelling, "Piggies!"

I looked out the window and sure enough, three large pigs raced by.

I went to the other side of the house and peered out another window in time to witness my husband chasing three more pigs across the yard.

Obviously pigs belong in a pen, not traipsing through the vegetable garden, availing themselves of an all-you-can-eat buffet. But, let me just say, when a three-hundred-pound pig doesn't want to do something, there's not much you can do. While Mom filmed from her back porch, laughing hysterically, the rest of us chased the moveable feast around the field.

"It's not funny, Susan," said my stepfather as his calloused hand gripped his beer and he lit another cigarette. "That's fifteen-hundred-dollars worth of meat running free out there."

The whole thing took a few hours— slop buckets dangled to entice them out of the road, three adults cursing a blue streak as Jake frolicked among them, making the job more difficult, until eventually we wrangled the porkers back home.

About that time, stepdad Bob decided there was a butcher in their immediate future.

DUN, DUN, DUN.

While I was happy to let Jake watch the circle of life play out from its inception, the death part of that circle was something I wasn't going to let him witness firsthand. If he'd freaked out about the mouse, albino frog, and turtle, surely the death of Daisy and Co. would necessitate a few therapy sessions.

We informed him in advance when it would happen and forced him to stay inside while the deed was done.

The deed itself wasn't particularly pretty.

Basically a guy stood in the middle of the pig pen, calmly put the butt of a shotgun up to the head of one of the pigs, and fired— then repeated the process seven more times.

It seemed quick and painless but watching them haul each one out by its hind legs as it hung from the tractor wasn't exactly . . . appetizing.

I felt so sad the next day when Jake walked by the empty pig pen, probably thinking about how his sweet Miss Daisy would soon accompany mashed potatoes and a side of peas on someone's plate.

"Mom, how much do you love me?"

"More than life itself."

"Wow, that's a lot, Mom. I don't think it can get any higher than that."

"That's true."

He was quiet for a few minutes, staring into the pen, and then asked, "We're not having pork chops for dinner tonight, right?"

I swallowed hard at the thought of him already contemplating eating his friends.

"No, honey. Not tonight."

"Good, because I'm not ready for that, yet."

These are the moments—the recalling of past memories, the wonder of life and its complexities—that keep me sane. My children are my reason, my love, my pride, and my joy. Whatever else is spiraling around in the cyclone of my life, they are what keep me from getting sucked into the vortex.

As for the other shit . . .

Well, I plan on exploiting *his* guilt as long as humanly possible.

Or until the guilt gets the better of me— whichever comes first.

I got the filter changed in my heater yesterday, three loads of laundry washed *and* folded, and he cooked the kids breakfast.

Am I proud of myself? No. But I hate folding laundry and making eggs. Let he who has plummeted from the moral high ground lighten my load for a while.

What I'd love to do is grab a change of clothes, call my friend and future partner in crime, Kat Nove, and saddle up for a road trip.

She'd amuse me.

I could count on her for that. Also, she has the one requirement necessary for this trip— she makes me laugh more than anyone else except for David Sedaris and I pay for the pleasure by purchasing his books. She does it for free.

Next, I want to do very bad things. I don't know what these bad things are yet, but I will start making a list as soon as *he's* finished mopping the kitchen floor.

I need to get in there to get a notepad and pen.

At some point, there will be forgiveness. I know that because I've been on the receiving end of it enough to know it's something you have to pay forward.

But not just now. A wise young man once said:

I'm not ready for that, yet.

Pig and Cow
by Jake Lopez

Pig

filthy, reeky

playful, enormous, starving

shorty, lethargic / mellow, tender

huge, spotty, patient

jumpers, cowbell

Cow

Obsessions and Compulsions

"Mom! Bring me the antibacterial hand wash!" Jake was having a moment. "Jaxson just put his hands down his pants and then touched my hat!"

Jake's a little touchy about his baseball cap. I'm not even allowed to wash the thing, and for someone with hygiene issues, this just didn't seem to make sense. But I stopped asking questions long ago.

"I'm gonna put my hands all over my butt and touch your DS!" he screamed at his brother, then promptly shoved his hands down his pants, rubbed his butt furiously, and then wiped them all over Jaxson's game, causing a fight.

Jake doesn't understand that Jaxson has absolutely no knowledge of germs. Nor does he particularly care about his DS being dirty. He'll sit naked, little wiener hanging out, in the middle of the living room, body dripping in catsup, furiously pushing buttons and sending little video game characters to all sorts of worlds, oblivious to the real one around him.

"Mom, he's not listening. He's touching me! Bring me the hand sanitizer!"

At some point I expect to enter his bedroom and find Jake naked, slathering his body with the contents of my thirty-two-ounce pump container of antibacterial hand wash.

I headed into the bedroom to bust some heads. "Jake, your brother does not understand about germs."

Balling up my hand, I knock on Jaxson's head: tap, tap.

"Nothing's getting in. Do you understand that? He doesn't get that you have a germ fetish. Just like I didn't get why you needed to collect mini-pencils as a child and couldn't sleep at night if they weren't next to your pillow along with your collection of baby dolls."

"I did not!"

Ah, the advantages of selective memory. But I haven't forgotten any of it— every obsessive compulsion they've ever had is burned into my psyche.

The pencil thing became an issue when Jake and his cousin Max flew to Michigan before we lived there, to stay with his grandparents for Christmas vacation. In my flurry of nervous packing, I'd forgotten to include them in his duffel bag. Once Jake arrived and realized they were missing, the dysfunction had metastasized across state lines.

Most situations I can fix. But hopping on an airplane to deliver his baggie full of mini-pencils wasn't an option.

"Great, Jen. The kid doesn't have his pencils. How's he supposed to sleep?" Mom was laughing over the phone, but two days into their vacation when she and my sister were forced to visit every Kwik-Stop and 7-11 in town to swipe tiny pencils from their Lotto displays, I'm guessing she wasn't so amused.

Another of Jake's issues is breath. If yours is bad, he'll tell you. Don't take it personally— he simply needs you to know that if you aren't sporting minty-fresh breath, he's going to need a good twelve inches of personal space, thank you very much.

By far, the obsession that was the most irritating was the Mad Guy/Sad Guy story.

Jake somehow got his hands on this cup that looked sort of like one of those wooden Tiki-torches you see at Disney in the Polynesian Village. One side had a mad looking face— the other a sad one. He'd carry it around the house and ask me to tell him a "Mad Guy/Sad Guy" story.

He tested my storytelling abilities daily, requiring that these characters occupy starring roles. After a while it was hard to come up with new material. Especially given his strict criteria.

"Okay, once upon a time, there was a man who worked at a grocery store . . ."

"The mad guy or the sad guy?" he asked. Jake continually interrupted the story for clarification, and God forbid the story took a turn he didn't like.

I'd lie on his bed and try to come up with something on the spot, looking around the room like Kevin Spacey's character in *The Usual Suspects*, fixating on any object for inspiration. "The sad guy," I said. "One day the sad guy put a video game on the counter for the mad guy to ring up . . . "

"What grocery store sells video games?" Jake asked, suspiciously.

"Okay, not a video game." My eyes darted around the room, focusing on an empty can of pop.

"Soda, he put his soda on the counter for the sad guy to ring up . . . "

"But he's a mad guy, wouldn't he *slam* them on the counter?"

Yeah, everyone's a critic.

"Okay, he *slams* them on the counter and says, 'Ring these up now.'"

"No, say it in a mean voice, Mom."

Not only did he critique my plot accuracy, but my acting ability as well.

"*Ring these up now!*" I yelled as Jake giggled and hugged his knees to his chest.

"Then what happened?"

And it went on and on like this, him interrupting after every line, requesting certain story arcs, dismissing any subplots he didn't like.

"No, Mom, why would the sad guy pull out a bat and hit the mad guy? That doesn't make sense!"

"Sad guys can get mad too, you know," I grumbled.

"No, not this sad guy. He's nice. Tell it right!"

Right, to him, was the same story over and over— the mad guy enters the sad guy's place of employment and basically torments him or does something to get the mad guy hauled off to jail.

"And then," I said, well into my story, "an alien appears outside the jail cell . . . "

"No, Mom, don't be stupid! Aliens don't show up at jail. Why would they do that?" His exasperation only fueled my desire to veer from the script. Call me horrible, but the more irritated he got, the funnier it was to me. Tears would stream down my cheeks as I lured him into the story I knew he'd like, only to smack him with something that didn't appeal to his sense of order.

"But wait, there's a surprise ending!" I'd get all wide-eyed and pause for long moments, watching his eyes fill with excitement.

"Yeah?"

"After the alien busted him out of jail, they caught him and took him to the mental institution because he was found running around the streets naked!"

"Mom," he whined.

"And when they got him there, they performed a lobotomy and he was no longer the mad guy. Now he was the slightly daft quiet guy that drooled."

"No, you can't change him! Put him back! Take back the lobotomy. What's a lobotomy, anyway?"

Jake has serious issues with change of any sort. This becomes tricky when you've got a mother who changes her hair color and style as much as she changes her underwear.

Once, while he was at school, my sister came over and put hair extensions in for me. At the time, I had black hair and after all was said and done, my previous chin-level bob was down to the small of my back.

To be fair, it wasn't a good look for me.

I looked like a Goth Wookie in red lipstick.

But it had taken her four hours to put in and, really, what girl doesn't want long luxurious hair to swing around and play dress up with now and again? I figured it would just take some getting used to.

So as my sister gathered up her hair supplies, I grabbed my keys and went to pick up my son from school.

Now, remember, when I'd dropped him off seven hours earlier, I looked considerably less . . . Wookie-ish.

As I sat in the car-riders line waiting for the daily procession of children to be walked out and seated on the sidewalk in front of the school building, I became one with my new do. As Jaxson watched a DVD in the back seat, I braided it, I put it up in a ponytail, then shook it out and pretended to be one of those beautiful women on the commercials who look vaguely malnourished and exclaim, "Don't hate me because I'm beautiful."

I hadn't even thought about Jake's reaction as I pulled to the front of the line and heard one of the car monitors call his name out after seeing it on the cardboard sign in my front window.

As she opened his door and he stepped up to get in, he looked at me, a strangled noise emanating from his throat.

"Go ahead, buddy. Get in." The car monitor gently nudged him, already looking to the next car in line and calling out a name. It was a very organized process and no lingering was allowed. Call the name, get the kid, shove them in and send the car packing.

"What happened to your hair?" Jake's eyes were huge and by the looks of it, he had no intention of getting in the car.

"Get in, honey. Aunt Resi gave me new hair. Do you like it?"

Jake slowly got in, never taking his eyes off me as I pulled out of the school parking lot.

"No."

"Really? I kind of like it." I smiled at myself in the rearview mirror.

"Mom, I don't think I'm going to be able to eat until you get rid of that hair."

"Well, then you're gonna get pretty darned hungry, my friend. Because it's staying for a while."

"How long is a while?" he asked a few minutes later, as we pulled into our driveway.

"Oh, a few weeks, maybe." I clicked off the ignition and helped Jaxson out of his car seat.

"Oh, man. Why do you have to make my life so hard?"

I Wonder if There is a Number One Pencil?
by Jake Lopez

I wonder what a Number 1 pencil looks like?
I would like to see what it looks like.
People always use a Number 2 pencil.
I think a Number 1 pencil is a special kind of pencil.
I'd like to see what a Number 1 pencil looks like.
I wish there was such a thing as a Number 1 pencil.

Raising Cain

My parents were hippies.

Back in the day, when they were still married, before they got old and turned from Democrats to Republican-Lites, they reared their children amid a gaggle of oddballs and delinquents— the house was always full, the laughs were always loud.

They tie-dyed everything that wasn't nailed down, they smoked pot, they sold pot, they made granola in the oven, and they smoked a little more pot.

My dad played the guitar and sang— my mother painted.

Together, they made me the person I am today.

As the skin on their bodies began to wrinkle, their political and moral outlooks grew slightly more conservative, as often happens when one sidles a bit closer to death.

Of course, they will both claim to still be Democrats, but that ninety-minute argument I had with my mother on Barak Obama's possible Muslim heritage speaks volumes. I was able to bully her into reason.

While I believe I might still be able to save my parents, my eighty-four-year-old Nanna is already a lost cause, bless her arthritic soul. Nanna says things like, "Oh, that Oprah. She's a pretty colored woman, isn't she?"

I cringed and looked around the drugstore to make sure nobody heard.

"Nanna, that word isn't appropriate."

"Why not? What's wrong with colored? It's not like I said the n-word." She paused to select her hemorrhoid cream as I shrank behind an endcap.

"Colored doesn't even make sense. Colored could mean someone was purple, Nanna. I'm colored. You're colored."

"So, should I be saying black, then?"

"African American."

"Oh for Heaven's sake, Jennifer."

"Well, I'm just saying. Black is a color, but I don't know any people who have skin that is actually black. Shades of brown, maybe. Would you say, 'That Oprah is a lovely mocha woman?'"

"Oh, leave me alone. I'm an old woman. I can say what I want. Grab me one of those boxes of Vagisil. I've got a wicked itch down there for some reason, though I can't imagine why. I'm not getting any action. It's probably dry rot. Your grandfather is useless since the cancer in his balls," she laughed heartily.

I have only vague recollections of my early years, probably because of the daily contact high or the desire to blot out painfully embarrassing memories.

Like the time my parents took my sister and me, along with the rest of their motley crew, to a theater to see *Young Frankenstein*. There I was, sitting on the aisle seat next to Rick, who was in a wheelchair, paralyzed from the neck down. The guy to my right was a big, hairy biker.

The lights went down . . .

All it took was Marty Feldman's name in the opening credits, and their hour-long giggling jag ensued. I wanted to die.

Today, *Young Frankenstein* is one of my favorite movies. I never said my parents didn't have good taste.

We rarely went to the theater, though, because the *drive-in* allowed you to pay a dollar for as many people as you could shove into a car and get there without being pulled over.

My sister and I were always put in the back, wearing our jammies, and told to go to sleep. We never did.

I'm not sure what compelled some of their viewing choices, but I do know that to this day, I cannot watch the movie *Tommy*. Seared into my brain are visions of baked beans coming out of a television set and some pitiful, deaf, dumb, blind kid, who apparently played a mean game of pinball.

I have vague recollections of my sister sitting on the floor, a Cheech and Chong album opened in her lap, sifting seeds from baggies of marijuana. She did a pretty damned good job of it, from what I'm told.

I have a picture of my dad sitting on the couch, a group of friends behind him and the biggest joint I've ever seen, in his hands. They'd taken advantage of the huge rolling paper inside the *Up in Smoke* album. On closer inspection, I can see myself in the background nodding off in a bamboo chair, just wanting to blend into the woodwork. My sister, however, is front and center, smiling and mugging for the camera.

When I was about ten, my mom decided to grow some marijuana plants in our backyard. A small garden was dug just under our large kitchen window— the pot plants up against the house camouflaged by a shrub and some flowers.

Those puppies got *big*! Mom would pinch off the buds and leaves and dry them in the microwave. I always prayed we wouldn't have visitors to the house on those days because you could smell the stuff a block away.

Until I awoke one morning to hear my mother screaming like a banshee in the backyard.

"Those little shits!"

I ran outside to ask her what was wrong, about the same time our sweet elderly neighbor approached our common fence, carrying a chicken carcass.

"What's wrong, dear?" she asked as she pulled chicken flesh off the boiled carcass and fed it to our cat, Mr. Rufus Bofus.

Mom was pretty quick on her feet. "Some of the neighborhood kids stole our beach chairs."

"Oh, that's a shame."

By the sliding glass doors were four empty holes in the ground— somewhere out there, a group of my neighborhood friends were having a laugh and a few bags of chips.

Sometimes I'm sad that my kids won't have the benefit of the childhood I had. There was a clear line between what a kid could do or say and what an adult could do or say. I don't think that's such a bad thing. We didn't turn into hooligans or miscreants. I've never been arrested, neither has my sister. We turned out all right. We might not raise our kids in the same way, but whatever they did, my parents managed to get us both through life fairly unscathed.

But I do want my kids to remember the stuff they were thinking and feeling, years from now when they look back. I'd like them to have the benefit of a trunk full of memories to sort through with their own kids. I guess I want to preserve the things I think they might forget.

From as far back as I can remember, I've encouraged Jake to write down his feelings. I now have a folder of notes, written in his own messy handwriting.

Notes to me, to his teacher, to Santa—the list is endless.

December 3, 2007
Note to the School Librarian

Dear Mrs. Schenk,

I know this is usually a fake excuse, but my dog really did chew up my library book called: *Robots: A New, True Book.* My mom said I had to say sorry because it is ruined and we had to throw it away. My mom wants to know how much it is to replace it. I am very sorry that I was not responsible with my library book.

Jake Lopez, Grade Four, Miss Boltze's class

December 2008
What Bothers Jake Lopez, By Me

It was a bad day. Things got out of schedule. The bus ride was a disaster. I hate school. I don't like gym. I had to go with another class. I did not act appropriate. I did not follow directions. Too many changes on Wednesday.

1. I am afraid I will say a bad word in class.
2. I am afraid that I will say I love you to my teacher and everyone will laugh.

3. Sometimes I shout out bad words at home about God.
4. I touch my private parts at home.
5. I have trouble understanding math.
6. When I get mad I can't think.
7. I play video games to escape my bad thoughts.
8. Sometimes I tell my Mom to shut up and then I feel bad.
9. I purposely crashed my four-wheeler into the wall in second grade.
10. I ran out of class in second grade when I was mad.
11. Dad spanks me when he is mad.
12. I let my dog lick my butt one time.
13. I don't like shirts with pointy shoulders.
14. I hurt Jaxson's eye one time when I threw my backpack.
15. I never lie. I have to tell the truth. I just can't help it.
16. I don't like the sound paper makes or the way it feels.
17. I hate people messing with my stuff.
18. I can't sleep in my own room because I am scared.

November 2, 2009
Why it Is Not Safe to Taste Chemicals or Any Substances Being Used in a Science Experiment

Because it could be poisonous and I could die. Also I could be allergic to the substance. Also I shold (sic) listen to the instructions my teacher gives me because my mom says he is not up there in front of the class talking just to hear his own voice. I am to follow instructions for my own safety. I forgot the rule and tasted the baking soda, because Miss Chipman told me some people brush there (sic) teeth with it. I will not put anything in my mouth in science class ever again. It tasted like salt.

I hope my kids look back and smile, just like I do when I think of my own childhood. I hope the bad mixes with the good becoming a wonderful stew of memories— I hope I teach them to make the right choices and when they don't, the consequences aren't too severe.

. . . hope, and hope, and hope.

I do know I wouldn't change anything about my own childhood. I am who I am because of how I was raised. For the shy kid who doesn't have a voice, having a bunch around you that are loud and diverse helps to fill in the empty gaps.

My kids have a lot of gaps. I hope I'm loud enough to fill them all.

Take it Easy

Jake got off the bus and whined, "This was, by far, the worst day ever."

Childbirth—the gift that keeps on giving.

But I'm working really hard on restricting my snarky comments to an internal dialogue. There were at least two words in my current internal dialogue that I didn't care to define. The kid didn't need any more obsessions—with his poop issues, the topic of hemorrhoids would venture a little too close to his hot-button issue.

"What happened, honey?"

Jake stormed into the house while I got the scoop from the van driver.

★★★

Jake doesn't travel well—he's sort of like his great-grandmother in that regard.

In a vehicle, he can't tolerate too much talking between the driver and passenger—usually my mother and myself. Because we often get into heated discussions Jake spends a great deal of time telling me to watch the road and telling Mom to stop distracting me.

Now we just don't take him anywhere when we're together, unless it's absolutely necessary.

Jake used to ride the big yellow school bus but after an incident in the winter when they ended up in a ditch, he won't set foot on that big yellow nightmare again.

Ever.

He had visions of the bus careening off a bridge and into water. I tried to reason with him—his bus route didn't even take them over a bridge, but he was not to be reassured. If I wanted him to go to school, I'd have to drive him, or he'd have to ride the special needs van with his brother.

An emergency IEP meeting was called where it was agreed that Jake could join Jaxson on the little van for the trip to and from school. That lasted for a while, until Jax went through a tantrum phase on the morning ride. This didn't send either child to school in a particularly good mood and was definitely not conducive to learning.

With kids like mine, if their day starts out bad, it's only going to plummet quickly toward hell. I happen to like their teachers and don't wish to put any of them through undue stress. They seem to appreciate that—and the extra snacks I regularly send for them. It can't hurt to suck up to the people who spend eight hours a day with my kids, along with six or eight other angels just like them.

I'm pretty sure they don't get paid enough.

Eventually I began taking both boys to school in the morning and they drove home with Dawn, the best special needs van driver in the world. Being the last person to have contact with the parents every day, the teachers gave her any information that needed to be shared when she dropped them off.

Let's just say, Dawn could write her own book.

★★★

"Yeah, he had a meltdown at lunch today. Poor kid. Apparently, the aid didn't get them down to the lunchroom before the rest of the little terrorists got there and the noise level got loud and concentrated around Jake and the rest of his class in line."

The "rest of his class" were four other kids. Four kids, each with their own individual issues— a bridge mix of eccentricities.

The noise got louder, the roughhousing got more intense, and five special needs kids lost it, in unison.

I imagine it looked something like this:

Jake began flapping his hands up and down, whining and covering his ears.

Christian started making nervous chirping sounds.

Sara got in someone's face and told them to *shut up!*

Cody fell on the floor and started banging his head against the wall.

. . . and Justin grabbed the vice principal's arm, demanding he be brought down to the boiler room to take a tour of the pipes within the bowels of the school proper.

Justin's "special interest" is pipes. When overwhelmed, autistic kids tend to head to their safe place— his safe place is anywhere a maze of pipes can be found.

What was clear: someone dropped the ball. Some poor teacher figured the six of them could make it through the lunch line without incident.

This was a mistake she wouldn't likely make again.

Dawn and I laughed out loud as she described the story. Over the van radio, The Eagles played— the irony of the lyrics not lost on me.

> . . . *Take it easy, take it easy*
> *Don't let the sound of your own wheels drive you crazy*
> *Lighten up while you still can* . . .

"Poor thing . . . " Dawn wiped the tears from her reddened face.

"Jake, or the teacher who had to deal with that hot mess for the rest of the day?"

This sent us both into another fit of hysterics.

Later, I sat Jake down for a talk about the day from hell. Apparently, the lunchroom fiasco hadn't been the only problem that day. At after-lunch recess, a group of kids tormented him and his friends, calling them retarded.

Yeah. It's moments like these, as a parent, I feel like a failure. Sure, I know all kids go through this, but all kids don't actually have a diagnosed disability. These kids know they're different, so every bullying situation, to them, feels like it has some truth in it.

I am not normal . . .

Why can't I be normal?

Will I be autistic forever, Mom?

Ugh. My heart breaks a little every time he says or asks something like that. I picture it beating inside me— comic strip band-aids holding the gushing blood in place. Snoopy covers the spot that took a hit when a second grade teacher told Jake he was "trouble" and then sent him to a chair, alone, in the back of the room for the rest of the day.

Banished. Singled out.

Buzz Lightyear taped over another break, trying to stem the quell of throbbing liquid threatening to pour out— the perpetrator of that one, a gym teacher who'd rolled his eyes at Jake during a Field Day race when he couldn't make it across the finish line with a beanbag on his head without holding it— sobbing his way across the field was how he dealt with his own shortcomings.

"Sweetie, I'm going to tell you a secret, but you can't tell anyone I told you this, okay?"

Jake looked up at me, wiping the tears from his eyes. "What?"

"But you promise not to repeat this, right?" I crossed my heart.

"Yeah." Jake crossed his heart.

"The thing is . . . " I couldn't believe I was about to do this, "Some kids are just stupid."

Jake's eyes widened. He knew I hated the use of that word regarding another person. I'd taught him it was inappropriate, yelled at him for saying it himself, and here I was, calling his "normal" bullying classmates stupid.

"But Mom—"

"—yeah, I know. Stupid is a bad word. I'd rather you say shit than call someone stupid."

"Mom, please." Jake doesn't like cursing. (How cool is that?)

"Okay, I'm sorry. But here's the deal. Kids your age, sometimes they're just stupid. Not stupid forever . . . "

Though, I know a few adults that will, indeed, be stupid forever, I had the presence of mind not to offer that tidbit.

" . . . but kids very often act stupid. Say stupid things. Saying you're retarded is stupid. Do you know what retarded means?"

Jake became incensed. "It's not good!"

"True. But retarded means not fully developed. A mean way to use it, like they did, means they think your brain is not fully developed."

"Is it?" Jake asked, both hands flying up to touch his head.

"Yes. In fact, your brain is just developed differently than theirs. Yours might even be better than theirs."

"Really?"

"Yes, and do you know why?"

"Why?"

"Because you'd never be stupid enough to call someone retarded."

He smiled. It started out a little twitch at the corners of his mouth and ended up wide, covering his face.

"That's true!"

"So, there you go."

I stood and headed out of the room, kissing the top of his head as I passed him.

"I love you, Mom."

"I love you too, buddy."

"I'm going to tell them that on Monday."

"You do that." I smiled and closed the door behind me, not looking forward to the kind of trouble Monday, and his truth telling, would bring.

Forget about that now, I thought, singing the song now in my mind:

> *. . . lighten up while you still can*
> *Don't even try to understand*
> *Just find a place to make your stand*
> *and take it easy . . .*

Journal Entry
by Jake Lopez

I don't like computer lab. There are so many buttons to push on the keyboard. I get confused with the buttons. I don't understand the Window button.

What is it for? Why is it there?

I don't like typing on the computer. I like paper better. My mom says I need to work on my handwriting. I write sloppy because my hands are nervous. I am going to try harder in class, but I am afraid I won't succeed.

That's why I run out of classes.

I run away from my problems.

I want to do better.

I will try.

The Decider

"Fine!" Jake fumed, stomping off to his bedroom with me yelling after him.

"Don't you dare walk away when I'm speaking to you. Get back—"

Slam.

Oh, no you didn't!

"Uh-oh . . . " his father said, with a bit too much humor in his voice for my good taste— not to mention my rising blood pressure.

He's no help in penal matters. I am the disciplinarian in the house. While he's the guy who brings home the bacon—and often chases the live versions around the yard—he also brings home fists full of cavity-creating candy, and I'm the gal left to worry over impending dental work. Or lack thereof, because neither kid will lay back and let a stranger poke around in their mouths with a metal object.

Oddly enough, dentists aren't particularly inclined to drug a kid for a simple check-up. So, basically their teeth will have to be falling out of their heads before any oral intervention happens. Their father, it appears, is working really hard to make that happen with his nightly guilt offerings.

To be fair, he works about sixty hours a week, so there's not much time for kid-play. On the weekends, though, when the option is there, he's usually out hunting, fishing, or hanging out with the guys in a considerably less responsibility-laden environment.

We each have our roles within the home. The good cop/bad cop routine might play well on fictional television programs, but here, while one of the cops gets to come out smelling like a bag of cotton candy, the other wears a whiff of . . . meanness.

I slammed through Jake's bedroom door, something I didn't usually do— as a rule I give him the respect of knocking first.

No, sir. Not today.

"Okay, buster. I want you to listen, and listen good." *Man, I was sounding way too much like my mother.* "When I'm talking, you're listening, got it?"

Jake nodded, frozen in place, wondering just how bad it was going to get.

"If there are words coming out of my mouth, you are watching my lips move. Understand?" It helps to be very specific and very literal.

Another nod but his face was still defiant. When his finger hit the ON button on the remote and the TV sprang to life, my blood pressure shot up a couple more points. I knew he could see it in my eyes because his own widened, considerably.

Danger, Danger!

"Please tell me you didn't just turn that television on while I'm talking to you."

"Okay, okay."

Oh God, this is how it's going to be throughout his teenage years, isn't it? He's already bigger than me, and he's only twelve. My job is to make sure he at least *believes* that I can drop him like a sack of potatoes if the need arises. I must continue to have the upper hand in this house or there will be anarchy.

"Disability or not, you will not be knowingly disrespectful to me under my roof, lest you find yourself with a packed bag, hitchhiking a ride out of Dodge. And Heaven forbid grandmother doesn't back me up, or she'll have a permanent boarder in her spare bedroom.

"When you're eighteen, feel free to walk away from me. Until then, I'm the decider in this household." It was out before I knew what I was saying.

Did I just quote George W. Bush? Oh, hell.

"In this house, I make the rules."

Jake stared at me through hooded eyes. "Why doesn't Dad make the rules?"

Good question.

"Your father isn't the boss of this house. He knows it, I know it, and your time here will go more smoothly if you know it. If you need one of your video game remotes fixed, he's your man. When I need the A/C filter changed, that's his area of expertise. Something electrical isn't working— he's the guy for the job. Consider your father tech-support. But I'm the friggin' CEO of this little business and everything else passes by my desk first, got it?"

I'm certain the tech-support reference went right over his head. It's a shame, really— my linguistic talents are being wasted on this family.

"When I get married, I'm gonna be the boss," Jake stubbornly replied.

"Good for you. That's just not how it shakes down in *this* family."

"Why not?"

I thought about it for a moment as Jake glowered, finally deciding on honesty.

"Because that's how he prefers it. And, frankly, I'm the better man for the job."

"You're better at being mean?"

Ugh! I walked right into that one.

"No, I'm better at getting things done. Keeping order, running a house on some sort of schedule, lest we have our own version of *Lord of the Flies* to deal with."

Oh, crap, crap, crapetty-crap!

"Flies?" Jake looked toward his window. During the summer flies often became trapped between the screen and the double windows, unable to escape. Death eventually found each insect so Jake had his own pet cemetery on his window sill. Because he couldn't stand to look at them, he kept his curtains closed year round. If he was waiting for me to get around to vacuuming fly carcasses from the exterior window sills, he'd be waiting a long time.

"No . . . " I wasn't about to let him veer from the topic at hand due to one of his obsessions. "*Lord of the Flies* is the title of a book. It's about a group of kids who, when left alone without adult supervision, pretty much got into a lot of trouble."

"What kind of trouble?"

"Tell you what. Ask your language arts teacher about it on Monday. She'll appreciate the allegorical reference if you mention it within the context of this discussion."

Again, right over his head. Why do I even bother?

His eyes went blank with confusion and, as if on cue, proof of my recent pronouncement entered and handed over a recently demolished video game remote, now back in working order.

Will handed Jake the remote. "Here. Don't throw it again."

Jake looked at me and I offered him a Cheshire grin.

See . . .

"Mom said she's the boss of you." Jake challenged, happy to call me on my recent declaration. Kids love nothing more than pitting one parent against the other— a universal symbol of spitefulness.

Will cut his eyes at me, one eyebrow at half mast.

"That's not exactly what I said. I merely pointed out that I run this house, and you just happen to fall under that . . . uh, umbrella . . . " The pseudo-master of the house shook his head, but said nothing. To his credit, he'd wisely chosen to remain silent on the issue, or risk having to wear dirty underwear to work for a week.

There is a certain power in holding all the cards.

The washing machine was my straight flush and I laid down my hand with a smile.

Gotta know when to hold 'em, know when to fold 'em . . .

Probably wondering why we were all huddled in Jake's room, the littlest member of the family ran in, his little brow furrowed. It only took a second to realize he was on a mission.

"Ma, camera where'd it go?" Jaxson put his little hands out to the side, palms up, and shrugged.

Holy Mary, Mother of God!

I looked from Jake to Will, and back to the eight-year-old before me.

I believe that was a complete sentence!

Correct me if I'm wrong, but I'm pretty sure there was a noun and a verb in there, accompanied by the understood question mark at the end, and a matching physical response.

Houston, we have liftoff !!

"Good talking, Jaxson!" I lifted him in the air and pummeled his face with kisses.

"Camera, where is it?" He said again and giggled as I set him down and began to search the house for his camera.

There is something miraculous that happens when a previously uncommunicative child realizes he's being understood. Things start to happen pretty quickly when they finally get that human back and forth has a purpose.

A whole new world opens up for them and it's like watching the Rockefeller Center Christmas tree light up. Boom! One minute everything's dark, the next minute all the world's aglow.

I remember when Jax first started school. He'd been assigned to a daily three-hour session for developmentally delayed children where they could assess him before a proper diagnosis could be made.

After the first couple of drives were over, I noticed he knew exactly where we were going. He seemed to be very good with directions, and from the back seat too. I could see him in the rearview mirror pointing left or right before I turned. If I took one road, he knew we were going to the store. Another road led us to school— and yet another, to heaven in the form of the Golden Arches.

Problems arose when he began using his own brand of sign language and grunting to direct me where *he* wanted to go. Needless to say, when he didn't get his way the car ride became considerably more dangerous. Screaming, kicking, pulling at anything within his reach— it wasn't fun for anyone involved.

I believe Jake's fear of transport began with the incident I now refer to as The Terrifying Car Ride into Hell.

Jaxson had been bad that day and as punishment we would absolutely not be stopping at a store where I knew the trouble would only crescendo to a mushroom cloud of awfulness. He'd want a toy, I'd say no, and then the entire Wal-Mart Supercenter would witness a full-on war.

Nope, I wasn't about to embark on that kind of drama.

Not today, my friend— the decider had decided.

So I headed home, and as soon as Jaxson realized where we were going, things snowballed toward hell pretty quickly.

"Oh, no . . . " Jake whined from the back seat next to his brother, knowing from past experience how this would play out. Jake promptly took a tiny size 4 shoe to the head. This caused my elder son to add his own groaning to the already explosive auditory experience.

Jax kicked the seat in front of him, sending my mother into the dashboard.

Jake wailed like someone was shoving a tuning fork up his ass.

"We're going to die!" he screamed, his poor face flushed, hair matted to his sweaty brow.

"Store . . . store . . . store . . . " the pint-sized imp choked out between sobs.

I tried to remain calm. "Jake, don't worry. Just stay calm. Ignore him. Mommy is fine. I promise I'll get you home safely."

"No you won't. You're going to get us in an accident. Please, Mom. Stop the car! I want to get out! You're going to kill us all!"

I'd taken many a sippie-cup to the head while driving, and while I knew I could maintain my spot on the road, Jake assumed death was imminent.

"*Oh . . . honey . . . no . . .*" said Jaxson. He'd recently begun parroting the one line I said to him probably fifteen-hundred times a day, and in this context made the situation more Fellini-esque.

There was nothing funny about what was going on as Jax continued to pound the passenger seat with his feet, screaming at the top of his lungs, snot flying everywhere. But, of course, Mom and I couldn't help laughing. I mean, once you venture so far into madness, the hysteria somehow becomes comical.

But Jake was being terrorized— a fact that became crystal clear as his brother took a handful of his hair and yanked mightily.

"Jaxson!" I screamed, "Stop it! That's not nice!"

I was torn between two children— one on full tilt, the other being beaten to a pulp by his younger brother.

"Don't worry about it, Mom," Jake sobbed, "just watch the road."

Oh, God. Bless his heart.

Poor Jake was being tortured, we were almost home, and I had two choices.

Option One: stop the vehicle and try to get Jax under control.

I knew this wouldn't work because if we stopped, he'd only point and flail and think we were turning around to his preferred destination, and since I didn't have a shit-load of duct tape and a muzzle somewhere in the car, option one wasn't going to work.

Option Two: Keep going and try to make it home alive, with everyone's appendages intact.

"Jaxson, STOP IT!" I screamed.

"Mom, pleeeeeaaaassssseeeee! I don't want to die!" Jake pleaded. "I'm just a young boy."

"*Oh, honey no!*" Jaxson wailed.

Mom was laughing and crying for Jake at the same time. I white-knuckled the steering wheel and calmly made it the rest of the way home.

After we managed to get the children inside, both taking to their rooms like animals surrendering to their respective cages, Mom and I just stared at one another.

"We're never doing that again," she said.

"Ever." I agreed, taking a much needed gulp of air.

"Really, Jen. Jake was tortured back there." Mom was sobbing now.

"I know. I get it. But I also can't give in to Jaxson all the time just to make our lives easier."

"I know that. But we don't have to take them out together if that's what's going to happen. Because I'm not doing that again."

"I agree." I was tired. Poor Jake took the physical brunt of the trauma, but I felt like I'd gone a round or two with Mike Tyson.

I don't mind taking Jax on by myself. I can handle it. But when he starts tormenting his brother, that I cannot handle. I have two children and I constantly have to make sure one isn't getting the shaft. To say that Jake pulled the short straw that day would be a vicious understatement.

The decider made a decision that day.

I would continue to push Jaxson to his limit, but I wouldn't require his brother to be any part of it.

It eventually paid off.

Autistic children often need to have their rigid sense of order tested so they learn what the rest of us already know.

Life is messy— it won't always go your way.

But it's one of those "show-don't-tell" moments. When Jax throws a fit, I try my best to hunker down and let him know who's boss. When Jake requires my sense of order to mirror his, and his OCD gets out of control in his effort to make things go his way, I point it out to him for his own good. He needs to learn he can't control everything around him. Sometimes he just has to roll with it. When I laugh because his social ineptitude in certain situations is bordering on being a sitcom, he's learning that's just who I am. From my reactions, he's starting to realize how other people might perceive him, but whether or not he decides to make changes is up to him. He gets to be who he is and I get to be who I am.

I will not censor myself for my children. Together, we're learning that life means playing the hand that we're dealt, not the one we wish we were holding.

February 17, 2009
by Jake Lopez

In the hall, someone was mean to me. She was nasty and rude. She was annoying. I hate her so much. She was teasing me. That wasn't very nice at all. I wish she wasn't at this school anymore. Or even this state.

She deserves to be in military school.

Then I went to the office.

The office people weren't listening to me. I got a little mad. They just ignored me when I came in. I didn't like that at all so I didn't get to give my lunch money to them. I wish they would have listened to me.

They are not nice at all.

So I left and threw my lunch money in the garbage can.

Appearances!

For the first seven or eight years of Jake's life, getting a haircut was a traumatic experience that must have felt like being tortured.

While I'm against forms of torture as a means to garnering information from terrorists, I have no issue torturing my own children for the sake of proper grooming. My thought at the time was that they had enough strikes against them personality wise, so issues like hair and clothing were a way to ensure at least the appearance of normalcy.

Appearances!

Early on, the easiest way to handle the grooming issue was to grab a set of clippers, pop on a two guard, and shave them down to the scalp. This accomplished two things— an easily maintained hair cut, and longer periods between having to repeat the process.

Unfortunately, the sound the clippers made was frightening enough to turn them into howling animals. They clawed at their faces as the itchy hair fell, causing welts. A fair amount of tears and snot added to the mix required they immediately be hosed down in the shower when finished, adding further insult to injury.

For many years before she retired, mother was a hairdresser by trade, so I had available to me an understanding barber with enough patience to finish the job. But trying to work on a moving target with a pair of scissors never seemed like a viable option. I envisioned two children with missing ears and gouged out eyes, and opted to go another route.

Haircuts, back then, required two people: one to hold the ducking, screaming head still, the other to grab the clippers and work at break-neck speed. The job was "done" when they began to hyperventilate, or a neighbor knocked on the front door, wondering if we required the services of local law enforcement.

For a long time, because he was even more aggressive than Jake when it came to getting his hair cut, I let Jax's hair get quite long, and only cut it when his vision became impaired. I even tried cutting the bangs and letting the rest grow, but a mullet on a toddler was not a good look and I had absolutely no intention of heading to the grocery store with a Billy Ray Cyrus look-alike in tow.

The first time I shaved Jax's head, I did it alone while his father was at work. This required putting him in a head lock, one arm holding him tightly against my chest, while the free hand shaved as much hair as it could come in contact with. Needless to say, I missed a few spots.

He looked like he had mange.

When I let him down out of the high chair, he ran to the bathroom mirror, saw his reflection and began sobbing even harder. He put his hands on either side of his face and shook his head sadly. This was the first indication that he might actually have a preference with regard to his hair style. He didn't appear to be pleased with the outcome, and to be fair, it wasn't my best work.

Believe me, I know all about bad haircuts. I've had my share. With a mother as a hairdresser, you tend to get used as a guinea pig. I've had perms that made my head look like a fluffy helmet, color that looked like it was mixed at a Crayola factory, and cuts that weren't meant for anyone but a poodle.

The thing is, I always bought into it. Sure, let's try purple. That'll be fun.

Perm, why not? Shag? Let's give it a go.

But my worst haircut, by far, was given to me at a hair salon where I worked with my mother. I was the receptionist, and about that time we had a group of interns working for free, learning their trade.

My boss was a "former" gay man, who'd recently seen the light and decided to marry a young woman right out of Bible college. Nobody took him seriously—it was hard not to laugh at someone who styled his own bride's hair on their wedding day because "it needs to look perfect."

He was less concerned with his sham of a marriage than having his betrothed look perfectly coiffed and styled.

Appearances!

Brian, a fifty-something gay coworker, leaned into me, coffee in one hand, cigarette in the other, and said, "Her hair isn't going to be the problem later tonight. Wait till that queen gets a whiff of what's between her—"

"Brian! Shhhh. He'll hear you."

"I don't give a shit," he scoffed. "What the hell is he trying to prove?"

"Maybe he loves her," I offered. "Can't people change?"

He rolled his eyes. "Oh honey, please. That wedding night is going to be a disaster. Mark my words, it's going to go down like the Titanic, but if that woman thinks *he's* going to be going down on—"

"Brian!" My cheeks burned with embarrassment, though I loved every naughty thing that came out of his mouth.

I was quite shy back then but that job yanked me out of my shell. You just can't be surrounded by gay men on a daily basis and continue to be a wallflower.

Plain Jane brings out the "makeover" gene in gay men, and I was his pet project.

Brian saw me as the weed Ralph Waldo Emerson once referred to as the "plant whose virtues have not yet been discovered." He was constantly coming up behind me, putting his hands up my shirt and adjusting my breasts inside my bra.

"For God's sake, get the girls together."

Oddly enough, it felt more clinical than an ob-gyn appointment and I reveled in having my own personal stylist around every day.

"What's up with your face? Where are your lips?" He'd ask, brow furrowed, staring at me.

"I don't like lipstick."

"Take my word. You need it."

Then one of his senior citizen clients would walk in and steal him away. Most of them were women who only had their hair washed once a week. Set and styled by him, they'd spend the remainder of the week lacquering it with enough coats of hairspray to make it last until their next appointment.

I can only imagine the horror of having to wash that crispy, week-old mess.

Then there was Jim. Sweet, anxious, twitchy Jim—prone to nervous hand sweating and bouts of depression.

When he was up, he was singing songs as Marilyn Monroe—breathy whispered lyrics accompanied by mini-dance numbers at reception—for my amusement. When he was down, he required a bit of coddling and God forbid he had a tricky client in his chair.

Many a time, Brian pulled him away from his station with a hurried, "Can I see you a minute?" then proceeded to re-mix his color to prevent an impending hair emergency.

The interns were a new way for my boss to get something for nothing. He was happy to exploit their talent, having them work for tips as indentured servants. They mainly shampooed everyone else's clients.

On slow days, they'd practice cuts on each other or on mannequin heads.

One day, I became the dummy in question.

Jim covered the desk for me as the intern we'll refer to as Meant Well led me to the shampoo bowl.

"I want to try a new cut. You up for it?" Meant Well asked.

"Sure." I smiled, ever the yes-gal.

I was shampooed, then led to his chair, silently hoping he'd finish before the boss came in for the day.

About halfway through the cut, I found myself wondering what look Meant Well was going for, but opted to remain silent. It's kind of hard to judge when the hair is wet and there's one long piece hanging in your eyes, obstructing your view.

At some point, the blow-dryer came out and he had me bend over while he dried the top. Immediately after I'd righted myself to a sitting position in the chair, I heard a loud gasp come from reception, followed by a frightened squeal. Out of my peripheral vision, I could see Jim and Brian at the front desk, looking straight at me. Brian was shaking his head, Jim had his hand over his mouth, and my boss walked in the front door, stopping dead in his tracks.

I looked into the mirror and gulped.

Meant Well had given me a flat top that stood straight up about three inches from my scalp. The sides and back were really short and a long, asymmetrical bang hung over one eye.

Now, I'm sure that cut would have looked great on someone else. Sinead O'Connor, perhaps. If she could pull off bald, this was a look she could probably handle.

The boss rushed over, glancing around the salon at the rest of the clients being worked on, then hissed into Meant Well's ear, "Take her to the back room and finish. She looks like a troll doll!"

He did—take me to the back and finish.

And I did—look like a troll doll—though I didn't tell the intern that. I didn't want to hurt his feelings.

"No, it's cool. I like it," I remember saying.

When I got home and my father saw it, he was stunned into silence. The man was used to some edgy fashion and haircuts from his brood. My sister was going through a punk-rock-ish stage at the time, my mom changed her hair with each passing fad, and he'd reluctantly been dragged to more than his fair share of hair shows.

But, clearly, this was too much. He shook his head, exasperated. "Jennifer, are you trying to make yourself look ugly?"

Yeah, that one stuck with me for a while.

Not the cut— *it* grew out pretty quickly.

The sting of his words, however, still have the power to make me cringe.

I remember standing there, a shy but impressionable nineteen-year-old, thinking: *I'm pretty sure Heathcliff Huxtable wouldn't have said that to one of his girls.*

I know he was coming from a place of concern— worried how people might see me with my shocking new cut.

Appearances!

I wished he'd handled it differently.

Like Brian, for example. The next day after my shift was over, he winked at me and motioned for me to join him at his haircutting station. He set me in his chair, pumped it up, and went to work. With a teasing comb and a bit of hair spray, he showed me how to fluff the once-eye-covering bang up and over to the side, rendering it a new hairstyle, instantly.

"There," he said, turning me to face the mirror, " . . . beautiful!"

Weeds are, by definition, any plant considered undesirable, unattractive, or troublesome, especially if growing where it is not wanted in cultivated ground.

I want to embrace the choices my boys make, not limit them or squelch their individuality. So, when my elder weed comes home from the store with his Grammy, having chosen bright yellow gardening boots adorned with pink daisies and matching pink gloves, I smile and say, "Aren't those lovely . . . "

Like James Russell Lowell said in 1848: '*A weed is but a flower in disguise.*'

No Children Were Harmed During the Making of this Film

Speaking of appearances . . .

Have you ever noticed how important context is to our lives? For instance, going commando—*sans undies*—beneath your sweatpants while grocery shopping: *Good!*

Going commando in a miniskirt for a visit to the local preschool: *Not good!*

Inappropriate context can ruin a mood, a great story, and in this case, a reputation.

It was a dark and stormy night . . . (actually it was daytime, but it was about to get really dark in other ways). Immediately after I hung up with the principal at the elementary school where Mom and I worked with the learning disabled students on film projects—the same school that Jaxson attends, I might add—my stomach churned, and at the odd occasional interval was accompanied by a violent burst of nausea. It swept through my midsection, agitating my already unstable nervous system.

The principal requested my presence in his office at 10 AM.

I heard Scooby-Doo's voice echo in my head. *Rut-ro* . . .

Immediately I ran to the bathroom and unloaded my angst. Even though I knew I hadn't done anything illegal, getting called to the office of the principal inspires the same guilty feelings as when I see a cop driving behind me. I immediately assume I've somehow blacked out and committed a series of heinous crimes.

I blame being raised Catholic. Being steeped in a strong tea of guilt and shame from a very young age does something to a person.

So Mom and I piled into her sporty Jeep and spent the entire trip to school wondering what he wanted to see us about.

Was Jaxson being thrown out of school?

Did they want to hire me to help at the school in some capacity, given how much the kids love Mom and me when we come to our weekly classes?

Which, I should mention was scheduled for 10:15 (. . . *was* being the operative word here. Are you beginning to get a whiff of some foreshadowing?).

Okay, so we arrived, headed through the office and waited for our appointment. The principal came out and invited us back to his chambers, making nice, shaking our hands, offering us a seat.

He said, "We're just waiting on the school superintendent to arrive. He needs to be here for this."

I still hadn't caught on, but Mom later told me she was suddenly aware of what this might be about and almost laughed out loud.

Then the broad-shouldered, slightly stocky but well-dressed school superintendent made his entrance. He shook our hands and removed his black leather jacket. I thought this was cool. If I have to deal with a school super, I want him to be the type that wears a black leather jacket. He got a few points from me there.

The principal began speaking before the super was even seated. "So, I guess we should start off by telling you why we're here."

"Great!" I said. I took a gulp of my large McDonald's mocha.

"Well, I think . . . the thing is, we can't have the school associated with anything where the word *porn* is involved." Super hesitated on the word porn as I choked on my coffee.

Porn? We were making a stop-motion animation short film with the class this year.

"Oh, nooooo," I heard Mom mutter under her breath.

"So we got some calls," Stocky Super says. "One was from *The Pioneer* . . . "

The Pioneer is our local newspaper here in Michigan. One that did a considerable amount of publicity for *The Bully Project*—the previous film project we worked on.

Apparently someone, somewhere, looked up our production company name and not only found my blog, but also my Internet Movie Database listing.

Essentially, every project we've ever done is listed on that page— my entire body of crappy filmmaking work neatly listed with clickable links to the video trailers:

Like that little gem called *Making Porn with Mom*.

And *The Bait Pile* which if I remember correctly included a trailer that featured my mother acting her dramatic ass off in the shower with a big pink dildo.

Ah, yes. And how can I forget *Macy's Wait*? The movie where I actually filmed two men kissing.

Still, I was pretty sure the word *porn* did it.

This was quite possibly the worst moment of my life. No, the word *worst* does not appropriately convey the feeling needed to describe this situation. Surreal? Unfathomable? Mortifying? Those aren't right either, but they saunter a bit closer to reality than *worst*.

Let's consider the *context* here. I posted a story on my blog that summarized the entire school filmmaking project and how it gave the kids the opportunity to find their inner voices and gain a sense of self-confidence. It was accompanied by a picture of the bright, shining faces of a class full of students on the night they premiered their movie at school.

Scroll down a bit and you'd find an unrelated blog post which was a satirical commentary on the dolls our children play with and how they look suspiciously like streetwalkers. Oh, and there's a cum shot. They're plastic toys and we used mayonnaise, but still. It doesn't matter. My blog had brought my personal filmmaking career and my professional one too close for comfort in the eyes of the school.

So, we were informed that in an effort to quell any more "issues" with the public, we'd have to sever all ties with the school . . . as filmmakers. They were still happy to educate my autistic son, thank Jesus in Heaven! Well, again, *happy* might not accurately convey their personal feelings at this point.

Production on the current project was halted, and the teacher we worked with was *suspiciously* absent that day as we collected our things.

I silently prayed she'd just come down with a raging case of the swine flu.

Returning home, my mom and I relayed the entire incident to our husbands, who both seemed mildly amused, though I'm not sure they grasped the enormity of the situation.

At that point my husband mentioned that someone from *The Pioneer* had called days earlier, trying to get ahold of me.

"What?"

"Yeah, they left a message."

"You didn't answer?"

"No, why would I?" the man busy putting new pine wood on the basement walls asked, nonchalantly.

The super and principal had actually apologized to us. They likened our creativity to Stephen Spielberg (I'd have preferred to be compared to Lynch, Aronofsky or Altman, but who was I to be splitting hairs?) and let us know that we did a great job with the kids. *No Judgment!* was positively seeping from their every pore. The meeting ended with us offering to give them all of the raw footage, sign something stating we wouldn't use any of the footage for anything in the future, yadda, yadda, yadda. (Mom, being the savvy producer she is, had made sure we covered our dirty derrières right from day one—we got release forms from every parent before starting this project. We still legally had full rights to the completed documentary and all of the footage.) But they assured us this would probably all go away, and they didn't need us to sign anything or give them the footage.

We left wondering just how much backlash we would have to deal with and if we were going to see our faces on the local news that night.

SMUT PURVEYORS CAST AN UGLY SHADOW
OVER THE FACE OF INNOCENCE.
STORY AT ELEVEN!

At that point, though, what I really felt was sad. Sad for the kids who had been so excited to participate in the project. Sure, I get it. I mean, if I saw a publicity package on some website, with my child's smiling face on the same page as the word porn, I might get a tad twitchy.

The whole thing left me with a raging case of the runs, but when clearer heads prevailed, reason won out over disappointment.

Unfortunately (or fortunately, as far as I'm concerned) I don't censor myself. In my writing and filmmaking, I explore any and every area I find interesting. Sometimes, my job is to put a spotlight on life's sores. So, if I have something to say about how certain popular toys look suspiciously like streetwalkers, and choose to do that through satiric faux porn, I'm going to do it.

And if I want to volunteer my time to help a class of learning disabled children on a project that helps them not only learn the art and fun of writing, but helps them gain self-confidence, I'm going to do that too.

Until such time as I'm told I'm no longer able to do that.

I am one person with many facets, each one as important as the other, and I don't believe one facet negates another.

For me, it's as simple as that.

Colors
by Jake Lopez

I like colors.
If there wasn't any color, it would all be black and white.
I like colors more than black and white.
My favorite color is blue.
I would hate it if it was all black and white.
Then I would never see the color blue.
I would be sad and miserable every day.
At least it isn't all black and white— everybody would be miserable.
I never liked black and white because they are very, very, very dull colors.
Who would like the world black and white, anyway?
I wonder if there are hidden colors in the world?
There might just be hidden colors in the world . . .

Truthiness

. . . the art of describing things a person claims to know instinctively, without regard to evidence, logic, or factual examination. A rhetorical device used in socio-political discourse to appeal to emotion, rather than fact.

Faux News, as well as other mainstream media, regularly dabble in *truthiness,* often using a menagerie of tactics to get their odd brand of reality to the masses. Some of these include, but are not limited to, using out of context quotes, ignoring facts, dismissing the messenger by preemptive attack, or the old one two: cut off and redirect.

Like the Nazi propaganda of old, a picture of total lies can be painted into a masterpiece of editing, leading the less educated viewer to actually believe what's being reported. When you can completely disregard fact and begin to embrace the idea that logic and truth don't really matter, life gets a bit easier.

For a few minutes, anyway.

My own foray into the world of *truthiness* came about after one of those parenting moments where you veer ever so slightly off course, eventually realizing you've taken a horribly wrong turn and can't find your way back.

Like the time I introduced Jake to the intricacies of armpit shaving by drag queens after being distracted by a Hooters billboard.

That was nothing compared to my newest faux pas.

"I'd never hurt anyone, right Mom?"

"Of course not, honey. Not on purpose. Why do you ask?"

"No, just say it. I'd never hurt anyone."

He's looking for a yes or no answer here, not equivocation.

"Why are you asking me this, Jake?"

"Because, I get bad thoughts in my head. I don't want to turn out to be a bad guy. What if I become a killer?"

Bad guys, to him, have always been the antagonistic characters in his video games and favorite cartoons. This whole killer thing has me troubled.

"You're not going to become a killer, Jake. I'm pretty sure killers don't sit around worrying about becoming killers. They just go out and do it. There's something wrong in their brains to make them able to kill someone. Normal people don't go out and kill people."

Shit. Now THAT was an inappropriate choice of words.

"Mom! There is something wrong with my brain. I'm autistic! Now I'm going to become a killer!"

"No, honey. You're not going to become a killer. I don't understand where this is coming from. Why do you think you could hurt someone?"

"Because I get bad thoughts in my head."

"Like what?"

I'm treading lightly here, and hoping he hasn't got a trunk full of gory crime scene photo-esque visuals he's working from, because I'd hate to think I'm raising the next Dahmer or Gacy. I've put in too much time and effort for that kind of result.

"I don't know. Just bad thoughts like I could be a killer and I don't know it yet."

Okay, let me back up about fifteen minutes, because my prior discussion with him leads me to believe that I've actually made his fears worse with one of my truthful observations, where a bit of *truthiness* would have been in order.

Jake had come home that day in a bad mood—something about Sara having made him really upset. He wouldn't talk about it for a while, and as usual, I gave him time to simmer down before discussing it with him. He didn't want to get into it, and so basically I entered his room, shut the door, and told him he couldn't have dinner until he told me what was bothering him.

The Wii was off limits as well. The video game is what I consider my "big guns" and I pull that one out as a last resort. It almost always has the desired result.

"Mom, I just don't want to talk about it!"

"Yes, I'm getting that, Jake. But it's important for you to feel comfortable talking with me about things that are bothering you. It'll make you feel better."

We sat for a long time. There was a fair amount of ignoring and staring, hemming and hawing. A tad of whining also played a key role, but when he realized I wasn't leaving until he spilled it, he began pacing the room. Clearly whatever he had to share was earth-shattering.

"She just made me so mad."

"Who?"

"Sara."

"Why? What did she do?"

"I can't tell you. It's too awful."

This doesn't sound good.

"Mom. Please. Don't. Make. Me. Say. It. Out. Loud!" Jake flopped down on the bed, covering his face.

"Honey, it's important that I know you can talk to me about anything. Bad things can happen when people keep too much inside."

He uncovered his eyes. "Like what kind of bad things?"

Oh, God. Really? Come on.

"Honey, some kids act out really badly . . . do really bad things because they can't share how they're feeling with their parents."

"Like who?" Jake needed specifics, and silly me said the first thing that came to my mind. It was a very, *very* stupid mistake.

Blunder, gaffe, miscalculation— none of these accurately describes how truly bad my lapse in judgment was.

Yes, folks, I told my autistic twelve-year-old about Columbine.

Well, first I made him promise to tell me his Sara story when I was finished, *then* I told him about Columbine.

A friend later mentioned I might as well have told him Hannibal Lecter had just moved in across the street and stir-fried autistic kids for dinner, accompanied by fava beans and a nice Chianti.

Anyway, I gave him the *abridged* version on Columbine, explaining the two shooters as bullied kids who had parents that weren't tuned in to what was going on with them. I even applied a metaphor: a pot ready to boil over because the lid was on too tight.

As his eyes got wider and wider, my panic grew in intensity, because I couldn't, for the life of me, shut my damned mouth. I continued digging myself deeper and deeper into a hole.

"But why would they want to shoot those kids, Mom?" Jake hugged the pillow to his chest, knees pulled up tightly to it.

"Because they probably didn't have someone to talk about their problems with. They just let it build and build and whatever was bothering them, they let it out in a very bad way."

Shut up, shut up, shut up!

"Oh my God, I'm going to be a killer!" Jake fidgeted, pulling a toy from his lap.

"No, honey. You are not. Because it is my job to make sure that you talk to me about your feelings so they don't get out of control. Now tell me what happened with Sara."

"Oh, Mom. It's just too horrible!" He was physically pained, clutching his stomach, kicking the pillow away.

"Just relax. I promise it feels better to tell someone. Don't be that pot that boils over."

Jake held his breath, his cheeks filling with air. After a few moments, he let the air out, offering his Sara story in one breath.

"She told Cody he had bad breath. She said that you stink, and she called some girl in the lunchroom . . . B–L–A–C–K." Jake collapsed back on the bed, covering his face.

When I didn't immediately say anything, he peeked at me through opened fingers.

"I've only met Sara once, but I'm pretty sure I wore deodorant that day. Why would she think I stink?"

I was beginning to think this Sara character was a little troublemaker.

"She told Cody he had bad breath. So I told her my mom said that wasn't nice to say out loud. She said 'Your mom stinks.'"

Oh, so it was more like—Your mom's stupid. She stinks.—That, I can live with. I'd rather people think I'm stupid than smelly.

And now I felt a tad remorseful for labeling her a troublemaker. She's another autistic kid—she's got her own menagerie of quirks to deal with.

"So, do you feel better now? Since you told me?"

"Yeah. But now I feel like I could turn into a killer. I think you should get rid of all of the knives in the house. And tell Grammy and Bob to stop hunting and get rid of the guns." Jake sat on his hands as if they were his own personal weapons of mass destruction.

"Honey, the guns are in a safe and only one person on the property has the combination. I'm pretty sure you don't need to worry about those. I'm forty years old and I've never touched a gun."

Jake's eyes darted around the room and he stiffened. "That vase could kill someone."

I looked at the large, phallic looking vase on his dresser.

Yeah, maybe if you shoved it up their—

"Or what about that TV? I could pick it up and smash someone with it." Jake was positively twitching with anxiety. Everything in the room was a possible murder weapon.

About now I was beginning to think that the Clue game Mom bought him hadn't been a wise decision. The first four games they played, Miss White had been the killer, and then Jake thought Miss White was evil, finally making Mom remove her card from the game entirely.

"Oh, Jake. For God's sake." My exasperation grew exponentially with his level of anxiety.

Suddenly, Jake seized on the toy clutched in his hand.

"Even this could be used as a weapon!" Jake tossed the Pez dispenser shaped like a snowman across the room as I pondered the possible ways to commit homicide with it.

Eye gouging? Shoving it down someone's windpipe? Pummeling by Pez?

Actually that sounds perfect for a dark comedy . . .

Wait. Stay on point!

"Okay, honey. Do you know what the word *irrational* means?"

Jake just shook his head.

"It's when you aren't thinking logically. Not thinking clearly. You are being irrational right now."

"Maybe you should tie my hands up. Then I couldn't ever hurt anyone."

Jake jumped off the bed, retrieving a skein of knitting yarn. "Here, tie my hands up."

Okay, so this was officially getting out of control. If I didn't think up something quick, homework wouldn't get done, I wouldn't get in the shower before midnight, and I'd have one kid who wouldn't be sleeping tonight.

I closed my eyes, thinking hard, willing something plausible out of my mouth— something that could put an end to this whole mess.

Then it came to me. *Truthiness.*

I took a breath and tried to summon whatever it is that enables Sean Hannity to do it with such ease, and so often— balls of steel, dripping with hubris.

Ignore the facts . . . preemptive attack . . . cut off and redirect.

Pick one, pick one!

"Jake, I just thought of something."

"What?" Jake stopped dead in his tracks, half a skein of yarn twisted around his wrists.

"I don't think there has ever been an autistic person who has killed someone."

So, sue me. I hadn't actually done any research. I didn't have any proof of what I'd just said— no graphs or flow charts to refer to. No visual aids or expertly edited footage that was associated with a story where it didn't belong in an effort to make my *truthiness* appear more truthful. All I had was supposition, weak at best.

Jake stared at me, his tethered wrists flopping down weakly.

"Really?"

"Really."

"You're not lying to me, right?"

Abort! Abort! Cut off and redirect.

"Hey, wanna order pizza for dinner?"

"Okay, I guess." Jake began unraveling the yarn from his wrists.

I sighed triumphantly, if a bit guiltily.

"I feel a little better now, Mom."

"I'm glad." I kissed him and left the room, heading for the phone to order pizza.

Truthiness.

It's not just for mainstream media anymore.

Sibling Variety

I assume my boys will one day have fond memories of each other and their forays into naughtiness—things that they'll look back on and laugh.

Recollections of tormenting me, or the dog, or their teachers.

"Ha, ha, ha, remember the time you covered yourself in petroleum jelly, then emptied a container of baby powder onto your bed and rolled in it?" Jake will ask his younger brother.

"Ah, yes. That was a mess, *n'est pas, mi hermano?*" Because in my dream, adult Jaxson not only speaks perfect English, but goes on to master Spanish, French and whatever they speak in Yemen, Kosovo, and Afghanistan.

"Or what about the time Max and I broke down the side gate, you got out and some strange man had to stop traffic in the middle of the road and walk up and down the street with you in his arms, wearing a stinky diaper, trying to find your home?" Adult Jake will chuckle, then take a puff off his Cuban cigar, flicking an errant ash from his silk kimono.

In my version of future paradise, Jake will be the eccentric Dog Groomer to the Stars, and take me with him on his international travels.

But, as someone very smart once told me, put hope in one hand and crap in the other and see which one fills up first.

In the case of my sister and me, most past transgressions can be attributed to her.

Resi—officially Teresa Ann Decker.

While I was the quiet one, she was the boisterous one—challenger of authority, blatant rule breaker. She's never been incarcerated, killed, or ended up on *Girls Gone Wild* or *Cops* but I wouldn't have been surprised if she had.

I'll now refer you to the High School Breath Mint incident in Resi's own words:

"My AP Chemistry teacher, Mr. Schmidt, was a real prick. I held an A average in his class, but still managed to get a three in conduct—three being the worst you could get. I remember Dad asked me: 'How can you get an A in the class, but a three in conduct? Are you throwing desks at the teacher, Teresa?'

"Any-who, Mr. Schmidt was going over some material at the podium regarding the periodic table of elements. I, of course, was chatting with Eddie Richards. Well, after about ten minutes into the lecture, Mr. Schmidt is suddenly standing at the foot of my desk saying, 'Why don't we let Ms. Decker repeat everything I just said . . .'

"Being the multi-tasker that I am, I'd managed to absorb every word while having my all important discussion with Eddie regarding that evening's festivities. So I started repeating everything he had said, *verbatim*. Mr. Schmidt says, 'That'll be enough,' but I keep going so he leans over my desk and in a very aggravated voice says, 'I said, that'll be *enough*.'

"And yes, I kept going. Finally Mr. Schmidt lost all composure and leaned over in my face and yelled, '*Shut up!*'

"I just smiled demurely and said, 'Really sir, please pop a breath mint.'"

This little vignette clearly illustrates the difference between my sister and me—I wouldn't have been talking with Eddie Richards in the first place.

She recently asked me if I remembered the time she'd pissed Mom off so badly, she was forced to hide under her bed and take cover. Apparently, I came into her room, stuck my face under the bed and said, "Why? Why do you do it, Resi? If you know it's gonna make her mad, just don't do it. It's that easy. Just be good."

I have no memory of this, but I was clearly playing the role of referee even then.

And I continue to do so.

Way before 9/11 and Hurricane Katrina my mom, my sister and I went to New Orleans for a frolicking good time that basically turned into a weeklong argument. I can't even remember about what now, but when we get together, that's just how we roll.

My sister was bound and determined to get some pot to The Big Easy with us, and after pondering all of the possible ways to smuggle it, she shrinkwrapped some, stuffed it into a tampon tube, and shuttled it vaginally.

This wasn't something either of us shared with Mom at the time, so I was left to worry my way through the baggage-checking process.

I kept praying there weren't any drug-sniffing dogs at the airport that would fly across the terminal and bury their muzzles in her crotch. But those were the days before all that nonsense we now call security. The flight attendants probably shared a joint in the john when they were having an off day. Now I assume they're forced to sniff ground-up hydrocodone tablets before they board in order to deal with a cabin full of mouth-breathing idiots who need a complimentary pillow and blanket for an hour-and-a-half flight. Fine by me. As long as the pilot isn't under the influence, the flight attendant staff can be hallucinating on mushrooms for all I care.

Now you can't even pack six ounces of shampoo in your luggage without being put on some terrorist watch list. And I'm not sure what kind of homicidal intent could be attributed to fingernail clippers, but I guess if you're crazy enough to kill someone, you can do it with anything, anywhere.

My sister is a veritable feast of memories that I've somehow managed to push deep into the recesses of my subconscious. My sister and mother have always had a contentious relationship. They're too much alike to be in the same room for any length of time, and in the past—before I started using my words to tell them both to shut the hell up—I'd end up stuck in the middle of every argument, trying to be the peacemaker.

On the New Orleans vacation, my sister didn't have much money, so my mother and I chipped in so she could come. This irritated my mother, but her ire didn't come out till later—when my sister ran down to five dollars on the *Queen of New Orleans* riverboat gambling cruise. She started hitting the free drinks while Mom and I were playing the slots. Just as we were all getting low on funds, Resi decided to spend her last five dollar bill at the blackjack table. By the time Mom and I sidled up to the table, Resi had doubled down (frequently) and was up $220 bucks.

Instead of being happy for her, Mom's eyes narrowed to slits. I imagine the reason Mom got so mad was because her youngest daughter, no matter how bad her decisions, always managed to land on two feet. While the rest of us tend to play it safe—get car insurance, mammograms, change the batteries in the fire alarms—Resi flies by the seat of her pricey undies and always makes it out unscathed. So her daughter having won enough cash to get through a trip she'd originally come into empty-handed, probably chapped Mom's ass. They spent the rest of the trip sniping at one another— I spent the rest of the trip with a case of anxiety hives.

"Oh! Don't forget to tell them about the time I was living with you and your first husband, and the Colombian Drug Lord named Jorge with the multiple beepers and phones came to pick me up in his Trans-Am to go to Miami for the weekend," Resi reminded me in an email.

Yeah, that was a precious moment I'd sooner forget. It wasn't till later that I found out her weekend involved a Santeria goat sacrifice and sleeping with a 9mm under her pillow in a $550 a night hotel suite.

What I did know was that a guy looking suspiciously like Al Pacino's character in *Scarface* came to pick her up, and she cheerfully left carrying her overnight bag as my stomach lurched somewhere into my bowels.

I was on the toilet all night, yelling to my first husband in the other room.

"He could just be a beeper salesman, right?"

"Jen," offered the guy raised in New York, "That guy was a drug dealer. Your sister is an idiot."

"Yeah, but some drug dealers can be nice, right?" I clutched my stomach and let loose with a river of effluent.

"Uh, huh. Sure." he offered, rolling over and turning out the bedside light.

Resi is a cat who's already lived eight of her nine lives, and now has the battle scars, in the form of anxiety attacks, high blood pressure and OCD to prove it.

"Ooh, don't forget to tell the story of my old boss at the strip club—the ex-DEA cop who shot his gun two inches from my head in his office at the club because his girlfriend left work early and I didn't tell him. That's a fun one, too."

Clearly, her idea of fun split from mine somewhere along the line—like at conception.

As the hair and makeup girl to the strippers, Resi spent a few years being the only person wearing clothes in a sea of t-backs and titty-tape. I have a faint recollection of her rushing one of the girls to the emergency room after she overdosed one night. What a sparkling memory that must be for her— the bright lights of the ER set against the backdrop of a scantily clad dancer being force-fed activated charcoal before having the contents of her stomach take a u-turn into an emesis basin.

Good times.

Resi once flirted herself out of a field sobriety test with a test-tube-shaped shot glass clearly visible between her breasts. I think the Victoria's Secret push-up bra helped because the cop gave her a wink and a verbal warning.

"Or you, Becky, and Debbie with the dookie-rolls and two cans of Aqua Net before any party nights in Apopka . . ."

Okay, that one's going way back, and not as perilous a memory. Back to high school and the days of big, crunchy hair. We'd hot roll our entire head, shake it out, stand in front of a fan, and apply a noxious amount of the strongest hairspray available in the free world. The outcome was hair that stood out from our ears a good six inches, and a "dookie-roll," or curled bang, that looked like it'd been set with a beer can.

This fashion faux pas resulted in a series of yearbook pictures I now call the Tammy Faye triptych.

We'd drive around town in my first car, an old 1970-something black Cadillac—the car you'd want your kid to be in if they were involved in an accident going seventy-five miles an hour. The thing was a tank.

If I'd put American flags on each corner of its hood, I could easily have been mistaken for the visiting POTUS. Man, we could cram some people in that puppy. Six could fit in the back seat and five in the front. Of course, I was always the official designated driver. Many nights I drove kids home who'd reward me by puking out the windows or on the back seat.

Once I dropped my sister off at a party, ran up to the store to get myself a nonalcoholic drink, and returned to find her funneling beer on the front lawn with a group of football players. That was the first year she joined me in high school and my popularity rating skyrocketed simply because she was my sister.

On that night, Resi was one of the pukers in question. I remember staying up all night listening to her retch into the toilet and hoping she wouldn't die.

While I don't want the memories my boys make to involve goat sacrifice, drug smuggling, Aqua Net or overdosing strippers, I do hope they can look back and smile one day—and if one of them is unable to remember a particularly funny story, hopefully the other will be able to fill in the gaps.

Nice Hands, Nice Feet, Nice Head, Nice Mouth

Jax got off the school van one day, extremely disturbed.

Normally, he'd immediately remove his jacket, shoes, and every other stitch of clothing except his undies. This time, he ran to my bed and lay down, fully clothed.

"Come 'ere," he requested, pulling my hand.

I lay down with him, hugging him to me and kissing his forehead.

"No kisses," he said, smacking his forehead where I'd just planted the kiss.

"What's wrong?" I asked.

"No what's wrong . . . " he whined, kicking his feet against me.

"It's okay . . . ," I soothed.

"No. No okay. Stuck . . . I sad."

Stuck, in Jaxson's case, refers to how he feels when he's restrained. When he becomes aggressive—hitting, kicking, head-butting, I have to hold him down as best I can without hurting him.

When I do this, he says, "Stuck."

Sensory-wise, he likes deep, firm pressure, so at school the teachers often roll a big yoga ball over his body, using their weight to sandwich him between the floor and the ball. He loves this. Many autistic people like firm pressure. It enables them to feel more "in their body." Like being anchored.

But he does not like being restrained—his body tells him the difference between the two.

His frustration, I learned after reading his journal as well as the incident report, was because he'd had another aggressive day and had to be restrained. Often, it takes two or three teachers— one holding his feet at the ankles, one holding his head, because he's prone to head-butting, and one at his chest.

They say to him, "Nice hands, nice feet, nice head, nice mouth."

Translation: no hitting, no kicking, no head-butting, no biting.

He must repeat this before he is able to get up. Compliance is important, so that they know he understands what they're asking. Twice this same week, Jaxson had become aggressive with staff. He pulled Mr. W's hair while being restrained once, and on another day, he managed to bust his teacher's lip by head-butting her.

The staff is used to this type of behavior, though Jaxson is probably the most aggressive in his particular class, and the restraint is for his safety as well as the safety of the other students. When Jax doesn't want to follow his schedule, provided on laminated cards with pictures that represent visual cues, he begins grabbing posters from the walls, tosses the bean bag chair around the room, and throws anything he can get his hands on.

The key is figuring out why he gets keyed up in the first place. It comes out of nowhere and then can disappear just as quickly with a smile on his face. Because he's not very verbal yet, he can't articulate what's bothering him.

Are the lights too bright?

Do you feel sick?

Are you confused, sad, mad, disappointed, frustrated?

His teacher said once, "I wish he came with a little USB port so we could plug him into the computer and find out what was going on in there."

So far, I've had little luck with the five different medicine combinations his pediatrician has tried. In Jaxson's case, it's also a behavioral issue. He's stubborn.

Stubborn and autistic is a menacing combo.

Some verbal autistic persons who have had aggression problems in the past have described this overwhelming anger that comes out of nowhere and is almost impossible to contain. One young man called it the werewolf in him coming out.

On that particular day, after I got Jaxson calmed down, he undressed and smiled, letting me know he was under control. With a little attention from me, he'd pulled it together and been able to self-calm.

I entered the kitchen about the time he turned on the television and said, "Egg san-wich. Catsup. Please."

Oh, how cute. He's getting so much better at his verbal communication! That was my first thought.

My second thought was: *Oh shit. I'm out of eggs.*

I knew this was the recipe for the perfect storm. Fresh from one fit, he'd slide into another, simply because I had no eggs in the house. He'd very calmly asked for an egg sandwich, like he was supposed to do when he wanted something. He'd done his part.

I'd be unable to do mine.

"Honey, I don't have any eggs."

I saw it in his eyes as he lowered his brow. Looking like Cro-Magnon man, he stared at me from underneath. He walked to the refrigerator, opened it, looked inside, then closed the refrigerator door.

Then he began to cry. Real tears, real sobbing. He approached me, looking toward the ceiling as he balled up his little fists and shook them toward the heavens.

"I can't take it anymore!" It was perfectly articulated.

My arms went around him and I chuckled before bending to whisper in his ear.

"It's okay."

"No, it's not okay," he sobbed. "I sad."

Okay, that's it. The kid was sad and I was bound and determined to get him what he wanted.

The eggs had simply been the period at the end of the sentence that was his horrible day, and if he wanted a damned egg sandwich, he'd be getting a damned egg sandwich. Sure, I knew I could redirect him— offer other viable food options and maybe even get away with it, *sans* tantrum. But the poor kid had been through the mill at school already. I think it's important, when I can, to provide the feeling of a safe-space for my children so they aren't constantly being barraged with demands and redirection.

Sometimes, a person just *needs* an egg sandwich— I know all about comfort food, believe me.

"Jake!" I yelled, "Can you come here, please?"

I'd enlist his big brother in my problem solving because leaving Jaxson alone in the house, even for five minutes, was not an option.

Much damage could be done in five minutes, especially when his mood was tenuous.

Jake shuffled out of his room. "Yeah?"

"I need you to do me a favor. I'm out of eggs and your brother wants an egg sandwich. Go over to the barn and see if there are any eggs in the fridge and if there aren't, go into the chicken coop and pull some from under their feathery behinds."

Interestingly, Jake doesn't mind retrieving eggs. He's more concerned with being pecked to death by chickens than the fact the eggs come out of their butts.

"Can I get paid?" Jake asked, tapping his foot.

"Check my purse and see how many singles I have."

I bent down to tell Jaxson, "Jake's going to go get some eggs, okay?"

Jax looked slightly confused. "Egg sandwich?"

"Yep, just a minute and I'll make you an egg sandwich." I kissed him on the top of his head.

"Yeah! Egg sandwich! Good job!" Jax hopped across the room to watch cartoons.

"You've got three dollars, Mom. Is it worth three dollars?"

"You betcha."

Jake headed out to the barn. I prayed the chickens didn't give him any trouble—this whole scenario could go horribly wrong if the chickens weren't compliant, and restraining *them* wouldn't work. They didn't respond to "nice claws, nice beak."

Five minutes later, with a carton of brown eggs fresh from the fowl derrières in hand, Jake returned with a smile, happy to be of service.

"Can I have some eggs, too?"

"Certainly," I said, popping the bread out of the toaster oven.

"I want mine over easy. Nothing else with them."

"Okay." I scrambled up a couple for Jax and tossed in another two for Jake, sunny-side up.

"Please don't put anything else on the plate, Mom. I like my food neat."

"What does that mean?" I cracked four eggs into the pan and tossed the shells into the slop bucket.

"Like touching each other. That's not acceptable. I like all of the food in their own groups, alone. I want them to go into my stomach neat, not in a big mess."

Oh, brother.

"Okay, I can handle that. Two eggs, neat. Coming up."

Jake headed to his room, turning abruptly as I flipped the eggs, trying not to break the yolks, as this would most certainly be problem scenario number two. Broken yolks can't stare at him sunny-side up.

"Mom . . . ," he whined quietly.

I waited for the other shoe to drop. In this house, there's always another damned shoe, and it's never Prada, by the way.

"Did you vacuum up the dead flies on my windowsill yet?"

"Jake . . . " There was a warning note in my voice, set against the backdrop of frying eggs.

"Mom, I can't eat in there with those dead flies. Please vacuum them up before I eat."

I shot him a sideways glance as I squirted catsup on Jaxson's toast.

"Should I do this before or after I make your eggs and clean up the mess?"

He pondered this for a moment. "If you do it after, my eggs will get cold."

Uh huh.

Another issue—cold food was not acceptable.

"Would you consider eating in another room, just this once?" I asked.

Jake only eats in his room. He doesn't like eating around other people, nor does he like watching other people eat. His room is his safe place.

I could see the anxiety rising inside of him as his eyes darted around the house, looking for another acceptable place to eat. Nope, kitchen was out. He could see the chickens eating birdseed in my garden, and eating eggs while forced to look at the butts from whence they'd come was not an option. The living room wouldn't work because his nearly naked brother was in there. Obviously, the bathroom was out of the question, and he could see the pig pen from my room, so that was out as well.

"Jake, I need you to keep it together, okay? I've just dealt with one dramatic moment—I can't handle another for at least an hour."

"But Mom . . . "

"Do you think you can vacuum them up while I finish the eggs?" Stupid question, but I gave it a try.

"Mom, I can't look at them. How can I vacuum them up and not look at them?"

Good point.

"Okay, here's what we're gonna do. I'll give Jax his sandwich, and then keep your eggs in the pan when they're done. They'll stay warm, and I'll quickly go to your room and take care of the flies. Bring the vacuum in there and I'll do it for you. Can you handle that?"

Jake smiled, running to get the vacuum. "Mom, you're the best mom ever."

Crisis averted—for the next few minutes, anyway.

I gave Jaxson his sandwich, rushed to take care of the fly situation, hurried back to get Jake his eggs, and watched him as he entered his room.

Success!

No more than fifteen minutes later, as I finished up the dishes, Jax entered the kitchen with his empty plate, catsup smeared across his smiling mouth.

"More?" he asked.

Sigh.

I grabbed the plate, fired up the stove, and started the process all over again.

I suddenly got choked up—thinking about what would happen in the future when Jaxson wants an egg sandwich. It's my biggest fear as a mother—not eggs, of course, but the future happiness of both my boys. How their wants and needs will be met when I'm not around to meet them. I think Jake will make it. He's an odd little duck, but he'll trundle through life, bobbing and weaving much like his mother does on a daily basis.

Jaxson is another story. If his physical volatility cannot be controlled, I'm frightened that I won't be able to handle him as he gets older. One day he'll tower over me and there will be no calming him down while restraining him. There might come a day when I'd have to realistically consider a group home.

Even writing the words makes me shudder because calling this a last resort is a vicious understatement.

It plagues my thoughts, haunts my dreams, and it never goes away.

Problems
by Jake Lopez

When I get frustrated or people pressure me, everything ends with a slam or a smash because I don't want to hurt people, just things.

I am nervous about middle school and high school because I am afraid I will do something bad.

When other kids yell at me it makes me nervous and mad.

I feel like some of my classmates don't understand me.

When something happens at school I have a hard time explaining it to my mom because it gets mixed up in my brain.

I have a hard time spelling words.

I get hyper when something is exciting.

I don't like gym because there is too much noise and people yelling at me and head phones don't help.

When I get stressed, I don't know what to do.

I don't like it when people ignore me.

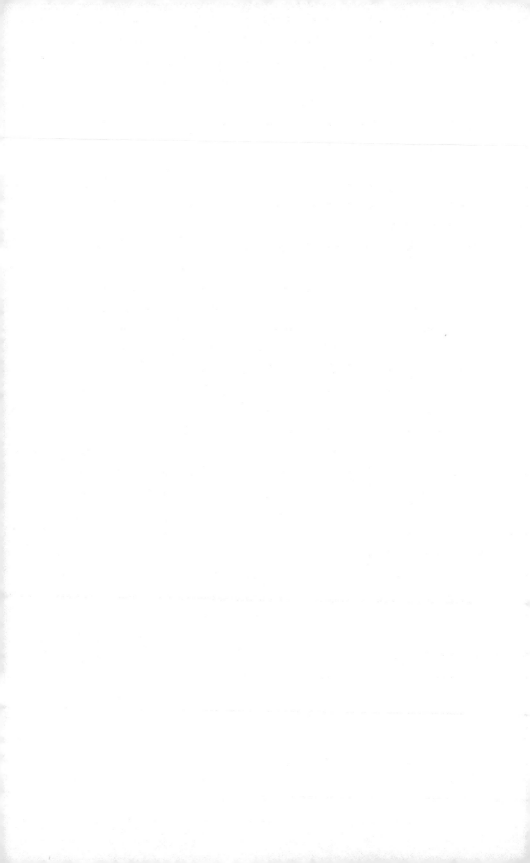

Santa: Give it a Friggin' Rest, Already

To a kid, it seems like an eternity from one December twenty-fifth to the next. I doubt I'm the only parent who feels like they come, go, and come right back again with unforgiving urgency.

Jax doesn't really get Christmas. He only knows that once a year, he gets out of bed and there are dozens of presents under a tree that we have, for some reason, erected in the living room. His look on Christmas morning is priceless, but he has no idea that every other eight-year-old he knows believes a fat man in a red and white suit left them.

For all I know, he thinks they magically appeared because he humped one of his stuffed toys the night before.

That would explain a lot.

At any rate, the fact that he doesn't even know who Santa Clause is makes Jax very easy to please. You can't be disappointed by something you aren't even expecting to happen. While the rest of his first grade peers spend their December days gluing cotton balls to red construction paper to make Santa hats, Jax just sees another day in art class where he can play with glue, paper, and scissors.

When he was younger, Jake seemed completely flummoxed by the Santa situation. He was more verbal than Jaxson was early on and would get excited right along with his fellow kindergartners, mimicking their behavior—but he had no idea what stringing popcorn for a tree and hanging up a stocking *meant*. Being a literal thinker, he had a lot of logistics questions.

What does the tree have to do with this Santa Claus person again? When he comes into the house, does he touch things? Does he use the bathroom, and if he does, will he remember to flush the toilet?

Those were the things he obsessed about when he was younger.

As he got older, and began to understand the implications, he jumped on the bandwagon, still not really getting the why of the stranger in the night, but happy to partake of his good tidings. Because the whole coming down the chimney thing gave his autistic brain quite the workout (we didn't have one), I had to tell him something that his literal mind would understand.

Santa had a master key that fit every keyhole in the world.

I was beginning to feel like a lying sack of shit—trying to explain flying reindeer and some guy who was rich enough to provide every child in the world with a pile of presents, even if it was only once a year.

He's autistic, not stupid. He doesn't have that suspension of disbelief factor that many children are happy to apply when toys are involved.

"Explain the reindeer thing to me again," he asked at ten years old.

"Give it a friggin' rest already," I remember saying.

"What do you mean?" Jake asked.

"Remember what we discussed about the Easter Bunny, the Tooth Fairy and Pokemon?"

"Yeah . . . ," he said, slowly letting out a sigh.

"Same with Santa."

"Oh, man." He slumped on his bed and frowned.

I tried to soften the blow. "Yeah, but you still get presents, so it's not all that bad."

It was all so easy before Jake learned the straight dope. But, once the secret was out, Santa could no longer be blamed for requested gifts that were not received.

Frankly, I resent the hell out of this.

Now that he knows he's got someone's feet to hold to the fire, lists are made, discussions are held, and lengthy Internet searching is required. It sort of feels like a list penned during a hostage negotiation.

Except for the requisite video games, Jake's Christmas list looks like something a demented scientist might have scrawled out after hatching a secret plan involving the destruction of the planet.

What does he plan on doing with a grappling hook?

Why has he circled listing # 3777 in the *American Science and Surplus* catalog, for a package of 638 2ML BOTTLES WITH CORKS?

Why would he need all of those tiny glass bottles?

Put them together with the boiling flask, Majic Air-Zooka, the Solar Rays kit, and the Van de Graff Generator kit, boasting 200,000 volts of electrostatic energy, and you've got yourself a recipe for impending calamity.

When I told his grandmother about the little bottles, she understood exactly why he'd need them. Since she played the same Zelda video games as Jake, she knew they were very useful. You could capture fairies with them, carry special water to make things grow instantly, or give a rock creature the power to break barriers. They could also carry fish food, healing gels, and fuel for your lantern—a must to get through those dark caves. If you didn't have them, the damn fairies would just flutter away.

What Jake was doing was preparing for his trip into unreality—the world of games, where he was in control and never felt different.

As I continued to scan the catalog, I saw another interesting advert circled: THE MAGNETIC STIRRER promised great functionality for use in the laboratory, but also "could be handy if you like your martinis stirred, not shaken, and your arm is tired after a long day at the lab."

Then there was the rock drill for $49.95. I understood the fun he might see in this. He is a boy, after all. Any kind of power tools are appealing, but this line from the advert gave me pause: CALL IT A SEMI-TOY THAT HAS TWO SAFETY LOCKS AND A DOME TO PROTECT FROM INJURY.

This "toy" would have to be kept safely out of the hands of his little brother, locked somewhere in Grandpa Bob's barn, along with the sword he was asking for, the "real Wolverine claws," bow and arrow, sling shot, boomerang, and blacksmith hammer.

Almost everything on his list wouldn't be allowed in my house.

What happens during the winter when he wants to play with something and has to hike down to the barn in six feet of snow to use it? I'll tell you what happens.

He doesn't.

He'll sit in his room playing video games while most of his Christmas list is relegated to the safety of locked cabinets, gathering dust.

I guess he'd enjoy knowing they were there for any possible scenario in which he might need to flay something with a sword, or pummel something with a hammer.

Or mix a martini.

Then there were the items he'd already secured down in our basement, so his brother couldn't get to them. His pots and pans, a glass coffee pot, tea kettle, wet-vac, an assortment of vases procured on thrift store jaunts, and a mini air-compressor because apparently he was assembling the necessities for life on his own.

A life that would include lots of vases filled with flowers and all the coffee or tea he might require.

I'm not sure what happened to the BeDazzler he requested a few years back.

I wish I knew. I'd have everything I owned BeDazzled by now because tacky is my middle name.

Then there were his prized possessions, relegated to a wooden shelf in his room built by Grandpa Bob: an English tea pot decorated with lavender flowers, his book on wildflowers, a gift he'd requested from his grandmother, and his collection of metal watering cans.

While I pondered the appropriateness of most of the choices on the current year's list, I headed with Mom to the local GameStop to purchase the pricier items.

Jake requested a Wii Fit. Now this was a gift I could embrace with glee. If he didn't like it, or quickly tired of it, I'd claim ownership and possibly work some of the fat off my ass. I'd also ordered Mom the new Stephen King book and knew I could read that when she was through. So that was two gifts I'd eventually be getting some personal use out of. If I was tenacious about it, I could probably think up a few more family gifts that would eventually end up in my possession.

As I handed over my debit card to take care of the bill that slightly resembled the gross national debt, I gave the boys behind the counter a piece of my mind.

"I want to thank you gentlemen for ruining my life, by the way."

Two sets of geeky-sweet eyes shot up at me, concerned about possible customer service retribution, via the toll free number given out on each receipt.

"Yeah, that new Mario game we reserved? It was wonderful to get an answering machine message in Mario's voice, announcing its arrival. 'Woo-Hoo, is'a Mario and have I got a suprisea' for youa.' Apparently, Mario is Italian or related to Chef Boyardee.

"You two know my kids are autistic. You've pretty much ruined all the work I've done to prove to him his favorite video game characters aren't real. Now we've got a message from Mario himself and I look like a complete idiot. He's listened to that two-minute message about fifteen times."

Both boys behind the counter smiled knowingly. They were actually great kids, who always helped us pick out appropriate games for the kids. This still didn't keep me from wanting to backhand them both.

"That'll be two hundred and forty-nine, sixty-seven."

Bite me.

That week, Jake spent hours printing pictures of swords and shields to show his Grandpa Bob.

"Jake, you want these made out of wood, right?" I queried, hopefully.

"No! I want metal ones!"

Poor Grandpa Bob. I pictured him in his shed for the next couple of weeks, pounding out scrap metal to resemble a shield.

Later, when Jake returned from the pole barn, he appeared dejected. "Dad, do you know anything about metal?"

Grandpa Bob must have informed him that he only had the appropriate tools to make toys out of wood.

"What?" Dad's first tactic is always to play dumb, because it has worked a number of times.

"What do you know about metal and welding?"

"Not much."

Jake grimaced and flopped down on the sofa.

"Mom, I need to do some more thinking." The disappointment in his voice was palpable.

"About what?"

"I am not giving up on this," Jake said with certainty.

As if he'd ever given up on any of his obsessions in the twelve years he'd favored us with his presence. I was still fielding questions about his

I Wish I Were Engulfed in Flames • 180

letters to the Nameless Yellow Blob of a Cartoon Character Most Foul on a weekly basis.

"What's wrong with a wooden sword and shield?" I asked.

"Oh, Mom. Forget it. Can I have a root beer? I need to do some thinking."

I nodded and Jake went to the fridge, retrieved a can of soda and headed for his bedroom.

"I'm going to my room to make plans."

To our credit, we waited until he was fully out of earshot before we had a nice chuckle at our son's expense.

It didn't last long, however. Jake came out within minutes.

"I have figured out an idea!" he proclaimed.

"What's that?"

"We could get some of that metal that you cut. From Lowe's. Then we could shape it into a square and then get a metal dowel and weld them together. For the shield, a metal top, like a garbage can top. We could hammer it out flat and cut it into the shape of a shield. That sounds good, right Mom?"

"Well, it sounds plausible, but you'd have to buy all of the supplies to make it. And I don't know how to weld metal. Welding falls under your father's job description."

I smiled broadly as my husband shook his head at me behind the stained-glass partition that separated the kitchen from the living room. I believe I heard him mumbling something about the *la apertura de mi boca grande*.

Seeing Pine Trees
By Jake Lopez

I
like Pine
trees. They make
me happy. But one day I
smushed a pine tree on purpose.
I will never do that again. It is wrong.
I still like Pine trees very much. They last
through the whole year without its leaves falling
off. There are a lot of different types of Pine trees in the
world. Some people cut them down and that is wrong.
If you want to decorate a Christmas tree, you shouldn't cut
it down. Decorate it outside. There are Pine tree seeds inside a pine
cone. I hope more people don't cut down pine trees.
They are important
to me and they are
important
to everyone else.

Pain in My Ass

I was sitting on a fluffy pillow, trying not to put any pressure on my lower extremities, or do anything like cough, sneeze, laugh or yell.

The previous night, I woke up at 3:38 AM, feeling like something untoward had happened to my lower back orifice while I slumbered—like a brutal ménage à *many*. Finger like waves of nausea and sharp pains filtered from my poopie hatch, up through my innards. I writhed around quietly, trying not to wake everyone in the house with my muffled screams of agony.

I knew there was only one thing that would properly remedy the situation, but unfortunately I'd let the tube run dry. I cursed my stupidity as I crawled across my bedroom floor and pondered the many ways I could efficiently kill myself should the need arise. The pain was unfathomable. Death seemed imminent.

During the delivery of my firstborn son, I'd acquired a souvenir that would hang about long after Jake was weaned from the bottle. In fact, my little *friends*—and notice that word is plural—continue to accompany me on my travels and travails in life—a tiny bunch of deflated mini-grapes just inside my anus, like a dormant volcano. Most of the time they rested and I didn't even know they were there.

Until they became angry.

Jake's birth had been a family affair. On the guest list: My mom, my mother-in-law, my sister, and Will's two teenage sisters. Also, Will was in and out because he kept going downstairs to chain-smoke. He wasn't much help in the actual process. He'd mostly just stare between my legs and get the same look on his face that he had the first time he saw a deer being gutted.

So, that's a grand total of six civilians staring at my hoo-ha during a span of eleven hours, along with the nursing staff at Arnold Palmer Hospital for Children and Women. Of course, the doctor made an appearance near the end, but I don't really count that, since I saw his face for all of about five minutes.

Then, presumably, he went back to his golf game.

Jake's imminent arrival, being the first male Lopez to spring from the loins of one of the elder Lopezes, was celebrated to the point of manic oppression. The sonogram picture was passed around to "Ooh's and Ah's," and the size of his little pee-pee was discussed ad nauseam.

I'd always wanted a girl to dress up in lots of pink and play Barbies with, but the Puerto Rican in-law contingent preferred the male children, my mother-in-law having had twin girls late in life. She promised boys were easier.

Girls, she said, were a pain in the ass. As it turned out, so were boys.

I don't think the human body is meant to withstand a three-hour pushing session. I'm not talking about three hours of labor. I'm talking about the *part* of labor where your knees are up by your ears, and you've got a mother and a mother-in-law, each holding back a leg, screaming, "Push! Push! You're almost there!"

I was sweating and wondering, "Why me?" and doing my Lamaze breathing, while managing *not* to cuss out any family members—which I consider a testament to my exquisite personality—when I heard Wanda, my sister-in-law, whisper, "What is *that*?"

She was at the business end of my body, pointing to an area that normally isn't available for public consumption.

"She's got a herniated area there," the nurse answered. What she was probably thinking was, *Man, that's gonna hurt like hell later.* I know that now, but at the time she seemed to regard my exploding butt-hole as one might peruse a fairly uninteresting newspaper article.

Both matriarchal heads popped down around my legs to, ahem, *assess* the area in question.

"Yikes," Margie offered, sucking in a breath.

Yeah, that's just what you want to hear on vaginal-slash-anal inspection.

I couldn't feel anything from the waist down, thanks to the miracle known as the epidural. I could have had a tribe of men hacking their way out of said orifice with machetes and been none the wiser.

A few hours later, I had a precious bundle of joy in my arms and hadn't given my herniated area another thought.

Until I stood up for the first time.

I did not feel I was exiting the hospital in the same condition I'd entered, that's for sure. I left carrying Jake, a few of those great baby blankets the hospitals have, a cool new formula bag, and a shit-load of medicated witch hazel pads. Clearly, the nursing staff knew it would be an issue, though nobody ever addressed it as they signed me out of the hospital. Not once did someone mention, "Yeah, by the way. Those aren't going anywhere. You will now and forever have a memory that's taken up residence just inside your booty-hole, lest you forget what happened here, today."

Be afraid. Be very afraid.

And I was, as I crawled on my bedroom floor in the wee hours, wondering if there was anything I could do to take the pain away because in two hours I'd have to get two children dressed and drive twenty minutes to school. That, I thought, might be a tad difficult if I was just having trouble breathing.

I lifted a leg and got myself into a standing position, immediately thinking I was going to faint.

I'm a fainter. I guess it's the body's way of shutting off when something assaultive happens, but since I was a kid, I've been a fainter, so I'm quite familiar with the warning signs. Instant nausea, impaired vision, and the feeling of impending death, all prior to lights out. I've woken up on the floor of the bathroom twice, one of those times managing to break my glasses in half.

What I did not want to do was faint, hit my head on something, and become unconscious while the rest of the members of my household gently slumbered.

Because the kids were sleeping with me that night, and Will was in Jake's room, I had no way of waking up my spouse and letting him in on my dilemma. I'd surely faint if I tried to make it to Jake's room. So I fell back on the bed, stretched my neck toward the fan, broke out in a flop sweat and thought I might vomit. By the time the clock showed ten minutes had passed—though it felt like six weeks—the pain abated slightly and my mind cleared enough to embark on a plan of action.

I imagined Jaxon saying, "Fink! Fink!" He'd picked it up from Jimmy Neutron. "Think! Think!" Jimmy'd said, his little fists balled up, his eyebrows scrunched together. Jax repeated it exactly, only he wasn't so good with the *thhhh* sound, yet.

I began to employ my Lamaze breathing for the third time in my life, trying to take quick, shallow breaths.

Now, hemorrhoid cream shrinks painful swelling, so what did I have at my disposal that might produce a similar effect?

Ice, I thought. Ice, might help with swelling, and didn't ice also numb things?

I briefly entertained the idea of crawling outside where a snow storm was in full swing, dropping my Tweety Bird pajama pants, spreading my cheeks and squatting onto a pile of snow. I could almost hear the sizzle of satisfaction that would emanate from my rear end. But I knew I couldn't make it that far. Just getting to the refrigerator seemed as possible as trekking through the Outback in the middle of summer with no sunscreen . . . or legs.

When I opened the freezer, I realized I had no ice. What I did have, were the freezer blocks, shaped like a soccer ball and a football that I used for my children's lunchboxes. For a brief moment, the idea of shoving a frozen soccer ball up my butt, then rinsing it and putting it in my son's lunchbox seemed slightly appealing. Believe you me, if it had been my only option, my son's sandwich, chips, and yogurt would have spent the next day in the company of a frozen soccer ball which had been formerly introduced to my sphincter the night previous.

When my eyes settled on the bag of frozen peas, I wondered what I'd cook for supper with the ham and potatoes because I was pretty sure I couldn't straddle my side-dish, then rinse and eat it as if nothing untoward had happened in the process.

Then I saw it. The long object seemed just right for the job—a lime green screw-on lid attached to a protruding six-inch plastic dowel meant to keep a sports cup cool for hours.

It looked like a frozen phallus attached to a convenient handle! The object in question said *Cool-Aids* on the side. My lower-forty tensed as

I tried not to laugh, snort, or breathe too hard—any of which would further contribute to the sharp, assy-treason I was experiencing.

I thanked God, Buddha, Allah, Mohamed and anyone else I thought might be responsible for my good luck as I shuffled to my bedroom and propped one knee against my bed for support. I bent my other leg at the knee and hiked it up like a dog peeing on a fire hydrant. Then, I leaned the frozen object into my rectum . . . *slightly*.

There was no insertion. I want that on record.

I pulled my undies back up to keep the frosty item in place, or at least as close to the target area as possible—and my entire va-jay-jay and pucker took only a few seconds to become nonexistent.

Blissfully numb.

I lowered my body to the bed and rolled on my side, the frozen thing jutting out behind me, straining my p.j. bottoms. I imagined I looked like someone with an erection protruding from their derrière.

The ice worked and I feel asleep, waking only when the alarm rang. For a minute, I thought it had all been a bad dream, until I stood and the now lukewarm, formerly frozen lid-slash-frozen-plastic-phallus fell down my pant leg and ended up on the floor next to the bed.

I got through my morning ritual in only minimal pain, made it to the store after dropping the kids off, and purchased an armload of hemorrhoid cream. Generic, by the way.

My nighttime pain wasn't a distant enough memory as Jax and Jake returned from school and Jake began with his question of the day.

"Mom, who's more likely to kill someone, me or Dora the Explorer?"

I tensed, then grimaced in pain. "Jake, I don't like that you keep asking about killing."

"It's just a question, Mom. Me or Dora? Who would be a more likely killer?"

That's it. I'm confiscating that Clue game from Mom.

"Well, since Dora is a fictional cartoon character and you're a real person, I'm gonna have to go with you, Jake."

I adjusted myself on my chair, putting my weight on my side, letting my tender area take a breather.

"I'm saying *if Dora's real*, who would have more of a chance of killing someone?"

I could tell he was deep in obsession mode: tell me what I want to hear, repeat it a few times, then all will be right with the world. I really wanted to prove a point, here. Get him to see that just because he bullied me into saying something, that didn't make it true. But I wasn't sure if today I'd be equal to the task. I didn't have all that much fight in me, given I had limited mobility, and laughter was not a good idea.

"But she's not real, Jake. What did I tell you about any animated figure you see on television with their own theme song? That's a good indication you're not going to be running into them any time soon."

Jax had turned up *Blue's Clues* on the television behind us and was singing along with the theme song. "*Now iss time for so-wong . . .*"

"Mom! Answer the question, please!"

I continued, " . . . any character on television that is a primary color—a color that a human would not be—is not real. Like if you went to Wal-Mart, you wouldn't expect to see Elmo or SpongeBob in the deli section picking up sliced ham—because they're not *real!*"

"*Fanks uh do-in you part . . . you sure ahh smaaht . . .*" Jax sang, climbing the TV table to plaster his face against the screen, right against the face of Steve the *Blue's Clues* guy.

"Mom! Please . . ." It was like an emotional tic. An itch that needed to be scratched—like checking to see if the door is locked seven times before he can safely go to sleep. Only this one was in his head.

I gave it one last-ditch effort, willing every muscle lower than my chest to relax and not clench.

"Hmmm. Well, I guess I'm still going to have to go with you. Dora's got quite the sunny disposition."

"I wouldn't be more likely to kill someone than Dora!"

"Jake, I just—"

"—You broke my heart, Mom." Jake slammed the refrigerator closed and glared at me from the kitchen.

This is where I experienced a bit of pain down south. The whole "broke my heart" thing caused me to guffaw. Not laugh, but guffaw, which is defined as loud, raucous laughter. Raucous laughter is not conducive to someone sporting an inflamed nether-region.

"Oh, Jake. For God's sake." I took a cleansing breath and hummed slightly, hoping the white noise inside my brain would distract my funny bone.

"That's not your true answer, right Mom?" His eyes pleaded for me to say what he wanted me to say.

"Jake, here's the deal. You asked me a question. Something clearly popped into your head and now you're obsessing about it. What you really seem to want is for me to say, 'Yes, Dora is more likely to kill someone than you.' Right?"

"Yes, say it."

"Okay, Dora is more likely to kill someone than you."

"Really? Tell me why."

Okay, I was gonna need a retouch on the lube job soon, and the veracity of the statement on the box—"provides prompt, soothing relief, and prevents further irritation"—was being tested. What I needed to do was let this one go and preserve my strength for a time when I'd be better equipped to deal with one of these conversations.

"Okay, Dora is more likely a killer because she's got deadly breath."

"Oh, that's funny Mom! I bet she does have bad breath, that stupid Dora." Jake clapped his hands together and yanked a package of carrots out of the refrigerator.

"What is your deal with Dora, Jake? Why do you hate her so much?"

"She's a stupid girl and I hate it when Jaxson watches that show."

"You used to watch it all the time when you were little."

"Well, now I'm big and I know better, and I know she'd be more likely to kill someone. I am not a killer."

"Have you ever seen a *Dora the Explorer* episode where she appeared to have some sort of homicidal intent?"

"What's homicidal indent?"

"Intent."

"Whatever. What is it?"

"When someone means to kill someone."

"No, but she has evil eyes."

"I see." I'd had just about enough of this conversation. "Can we talk about this later? I need to go to the bathroom." I got up out of my chair and shuffled, slightly hunched over, toward my bedroom.

"Why are you walking like that, Mom?" Jake asked, biting into a carrot.

"You don't want to know, buddy. Take my word." I slammed the bathroom door on my firstborn pain in the ass and prepared for the task at hand.

"Mom, are you going pee or poo?" Jake tentatively asked from outside the door.

"Don't worry, honey. There's no way I'm pooping today."

★★★

Since writing this, I've received quite a few suggestions with regard to hemorrhoids. I'm happy to entertain any and all ideas, including homeopathic, drug-related, Grannie's cure-all's, and folk remedies.

Recently, I was told a clove of garlic works—just insert it up the chute. Supposedly, it will keep the dog's nose out of my backside, as well.

Good to know.

Oh, Mother, Who Art Thou?

"*Jingle bells, jingle bells, what a crappy day . . .*"

I was about to be stuck inside a car with my mother and Jake, traveling in bad weather conditions, headed for Christmas shopping. The country roads we'd be forced to negotiate were icy and because we live near the ass-crack of oblivion, the snow plow hadn't seen fit to visit.

There were so many things wrong with the scenario about to unfold, including but not limited to Mom and I in the car together, without the benefit of a ball gag for her mouth and a handful of Valium for mine. Add to that the fact that my ass was still smarting, and you've got a recipe for a real hemorrhoid of a day.

The only reason I'd agreed to go was because it was Pig Slaughter Day-Redux. Our second set of little oinkers had partaken of their last meal and were now Dead Pigs Walking. Jake certainly didn't need to be privy to what would happen next, as six guys loitered by the barn, one armed with a rifle.

"*Pork rinds crackle on an open fire . . .*"

Jake was already in the red on the Obsess-O-Meter about braving the inclement weather, and I was lamenting the fact that I'd be at the mercy of my mother's driving.

Now, I love my Mommy Dearest, but I don't have the same faith in her ability to keep me alive as I did when I was ten and still believed in Santa. Mom is prone to losing her glasses, keys, cell phone, and/or anything else not tethered to her. Her train of thought also wanders away on occasion. This does not breed optimism, with regard to her driving prowess.

It had, however, given me a fabulous idea for a new invention.

The Senior Keeper-Upper: a Velcro belt with pockets and tiny attachable stretch-cords to keep track of phones, keys, eyeglasses, dentures, Life-Alert bracelet, and any other daily necessities the elder among us might require. Other features include a tiny GPS device, in case they misplace themselves, and a shock button, should the 'ole ticker need a jump start. It'll be a steal at four easy payments of $19.95.

Unfortunately, there's nothing on that handy-dandy senior belt for her train of thought problem. I've promised her that when she's slipped so far into dementia that she can't remember my name, I will remember hers— though I'll probably start calling her Gertrude and fabricating scenarios for my own personal amusement.

Didn't we have a lovely day on the Hubble Space Station, Gertrude? Well, yes I know I'm a great daughter. Did you enjoy dining with President Oprah Winfrey today? She's a lovely woman, isn't she? Here, let me wipe that drool from your chin . . .

When we trudged through the snow to the car, I could see Jake eyeing his grandmother suspiciously as she climbed behind the wheel of my Chevy Tahoe.

Mom had never driven my car, but Jake refused to travel the snowy roads in the rolling deathtrap she called her Jeep. Sure, the brand name inspired safety, but my knees hitting the dashboard in the passenger seat of the two-door sport vehicle led me to believe a head-on collision would leave all occupants in nothing less than a minced condition.

She acted all calm and confident as she turned the key in the ignition, adjusting the heater. I knew better.

Mom is a good actor and has been using truthiness to her advantage way before Steven Colbert entered the scene. She reminds me of the fake wizard at the end of the *Wizard of Oz.*

A flurry of lines filled my head, raining down like flakes on the snow-globe that was my brain.

Pay no attention to the woman behind the wheel.

All is well with the world.

'*Sure . . . if you hit something I'll be quiet . . . forever.*'

I was bordering on a panic attack and decided to distract myself by bastardizing Christmas songs in my head, rather than argue with my mother in the car.

"*Edna the red-nosed crack whore . . .*"

Jake fastened his seatbelt. "You guys aren't going to argue, right Mom?"

"Right, honey."

Mom smiled, pulling a tape recorder out of her purse. She pushed the red record button and set it on the center console between us, then pulled down the driveway.

Good idea, I thought. *My next chapter will write itself— I'll only have to provide the stenography.*

The rear end of the car jackknifed slightly as Mom made her first turn. She immediately informed me her Jeep would have handled the road better. I immediately rebutted by telling her that sounded like a blatant excuse for less than stellar driving.

"*Grandma got run over by a snow-plow . . .* "

"See, this road has almost no snow on it, Jake. Nice and comfortable and relaxing. I'm pretty good at driving in the snow." This was antithetical to the actions of her fingers, which began fidgeting with the four-wheel drive buttons.

As she drove a little faster than the fifteen miles an hour I'd have preferred, she rattled off questions to Jake, hoping to distract him.

"How many gifts do you have to buy, Jake?"

"Mom, you, Dad, Bob . . ."

I sat on my clenched fingers and wished they'd both just shut the hell up. While driving, Mom was prone to fiddling with her cell phone, her purse, the heater buttons and radio—all things that caused my sphincter to clench—and I needed to be prepared in case her hands started wandering.

"*I saw Grandpa fondling Santa Claus . . .* "

I glanced at the speedometer and noticed she was going ten miles over the speed limit. "You need to slow down, Mother."

"Mom, be quiet. Don't start arguing," Jake yelled at me from the backseat.

"Jennifer," Mom warned, and I could swear she pressed on the gas pedal harder.

"Don't push on the gas so hard," I hissed, gripping my seat.

"I didn't, Jennifer. The car is in four-wheel drive so it's hugging the road."

Hugging, my ass. Hugging is an affectionate word. What the car was doing wasn't even remotely affectionate.

"I prefer silence in the car. Then nobody gets upset," I offered, to finally shut everyone up.

"Yeah. What happened to the no talking in the car rule?" Jake asked.

"Exactly." Mom glanced down at the tape recorder. Suddenly it dawned on me that I was a worse backseat driver than my autistic son, and Mom's intent, with regard to the recording device, might not have been so . . . innocent.

Grrrrr. So, that's how we're gonna play it, huh?

"*No, Gertrude, honey. We don't shower anymore, as a people. President Winfrey has put a ban on all bathing. I'm sorry, dear, but that goes for naps, Regis Philbin, and ice cream. Now scamper on over and wash those dishes, and maybe I'll take you to Disneyland tomorrow.*"

We stopped and got gas, where there was a brief disturbance as Jake fought unsuccessfully to open the public bathroom with the key the clerk had provided for him.

His nervous bladder had gotten the better of him, only fifteen minutes into our trip.

"I want to do it myself!" he yelled, refusing to let Mom unlock it for him.

Thankfully, the door eventually opened and he disappeared inside to do his business, after handing the key to Mom to return to the clerk.

Mission complete, he sprinted across the cement, jumping into the backseat.

"Come on, let's go before the cops come."

"What did you say about the cops?" I asked, turning around in my seat.

"Nothing, just ignore me. I thought we had a silence rule in the car." Jake craned his neck, looking back toward the gas station bathroom.

"What did you do in there, Jake?" I wondered what possible shenanigans he could have been up to that might have required police intervention.

"I didn't lock the door back up."

"*Thhhhhht,*" Mom sucked her teeth. "Don't worry about it, Jake. It probably locks itself when you shut it."

"Grammy, don't do the teeth-sucking thing."

"*Fros-T the Snow Pimp, started jerkin' on his pole . . .*"

I took a deep, cleansing breath and pretended I was running through an open field, with daisies all around me— kind of like a sanitary napkin commercial. When that didn't work, I returned to my image of the snowman masturbating.

" . . . *with a corn-cob pipe and a button nose, and two balls made out of coal.*"

Mom pulled into a spot outside the busy shopping center and we all piled out and trekked across the bustling lot.

Clomp, clomp, clomp. Jake's feet dragged across the cement with the lethargy of someone wearing his snow boots for the first time that season.

"Jake, how about picking your feet up as you walk, buddy?" I begged, my nerves in shreds.

Jake took off across the parking lot to the sidewalk.

"Honey, don't run when there's ice on the ground. You might fall," I yelled to him, as Mom pointed the recording device directly in my face.

"Yeah, keep it up, Jen. On and on and on."

Just wait, old lady . . .

"*No, Gertrude, honey. Pink hot-pants are all the rage with the old folks these days. Now put on that sequined blouse I bought you and let's head up to the Japanese Steak House. You love watching those guys cook at the table, don't you? But, lest we forget what happened the last time, just remember: Stop, Drop, and Roll.*"

We'd only been in the store for fifteen minutes.

"You guys are stressing me out. Looking and talking, looking and talking." Jake covered his ears. He was being sensory-challenged by all of the lights and sounds and he wasn't feeling much like shopping anymore.

He was already thinking about lunch.

"Focus. How much money do you have left?" Mom tried to get him back on track.

Jake pulled out his wallet and checked his funds against what he still had to purchase. He picked out a toy for his brother, and with his shopping completed, assumed we'd be leaving.

Wrong.

Next, we headed over to the grocery section and braved the crowds as Jake became obsessed about getting his hand stuck in the cup holder attached to the cart.

"I'm afraid I'm going to get my hand stuck in there," he stressed, hand hovering over the cup holder.

"Then don't put your hand in there," I said, swatting his hand away.

Jake stared at the cup holder, shaking his head. "Cover the hole, Mom."

I spent the remainder of our time in that store, trying to push the cart while covering the cup holder.

It was in the parking lot, as we loaded our bags in the car, that Jake saw him. A man standing in the corner of the shopping center parking lot with a cardboard sign that read: WILL WORK FOR FOOD FOR FAMILY.

"Mom, look at that sign. Do you see that man?"

Yes, and I'd hoped you hadn't.

"Where do you think he lives?" Jake wondered.

"I don't know, Jake."

"What does that sign mean?" Jake stared at the man as cars continued to pass him.

"It means he wants money," Mom said.

"What do you think is wrong with the poor guy?" Jake craned his neck, eyes still on the man.

"I don't know, Jake. Maybe he doesn't have a job."

"I feel sorry for that guy."

"Sometimes people just do that to make money," Mom said.

"But he's just standing there. Can't we go talk to him?"

"No."

"Why? He looks so sad."

It went on and on like this for way too long.

"Didn't you see his sign, Mom?"

"Yes, honey. I saw it."

After Jake asked where we thought the man lived, how many kids he had, why he'd been fired, and how we could be so horrible that we wouldn't stop and offer him money, Mom presented a tiny lie, probably inspired by the fast food restaurant drive-thru we'd just exited.

"Last year we gave a guy some money, just like that guy, and later your mother and I saw him at McDonalds having a nice lunch at our expense."

Something about this sent Jake into a fit of giggles, which he continued for the rest of the ride home.

I was just about to give Mom props for her fast thinking when she opened the fast food bag then and elbowed the steering wheel as she unwrapped a chicken wrap.

"I'm really not comfortable with you eating while driving, Mom."

"I'm fine, Jennifer." Mom looked down, as if to ensure the device between us was still recording.

I stared straight ahead.

Oh Gertrude. You have no idea how much fun we're gonna have together.

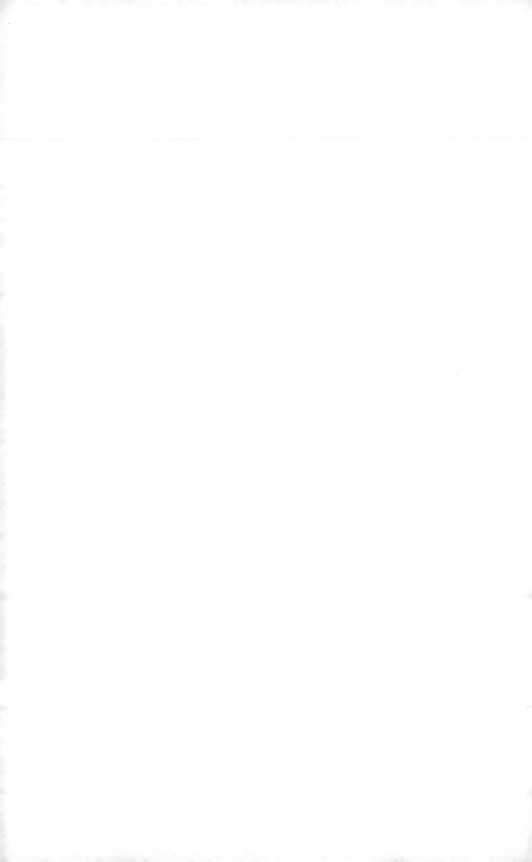

Say What?

I held the phone out from my head slightly as Nanna ranted. It had been forty-five minutes and my ear was beginning to feel like a pickled egg.

" . . . and my sister called this morning, Jennifer. Again with the accusations. She swears I had sex with her husband. I told her Mike stank, I'd never let him touch me. But she swears. She can't say when, can't prove it, but she swears."

"Just ignore her, Nanna. She's going senile."

Another one of many long-distance phone calls with Nanna, who regularly spat out a repeating rolodex of conversations she'd supposedly had over the phone with her sister. She and Auntie Toni would only rarely call one another because they constantly fought. Nanna was almost deaf, and her sister was beginning to experience some dementia. The combination of Nanna's inability to hear and her sibling's fuzzy brain was a dicey proposition, at best.

I listened giddily to Nanna's version of events, knowing it was probably a bastardized version of the actual conversation— one that might have started with a friendly exchange of hellos but ended up in an argument about marital infidelity. The getting from point A to point B, though, was nothing short of five-star entertainment. The added benefit, as a writer, was the knowledge that I'd work it into a story at some point.

I didn't necessarily consider this exploitation, so much as the preservation of their essence for posterity.

Yes, that's it. I'm an essence preservationist.

I scribbled notes as she yelled, clearly not wearing her hearing aid.

"Oh, she's not senile, just spiteful. She hates me. Daddy always liked me more. Sleep with Mike? Please. She knows I've only ever slept with your grandfather. I've told you all I want it on my headstone: HERE LIES CHICK WHO HAD ONLY ONE DICK."

Here Lies Chick . . . I scribbled. I'd heard that one numerous times over the years. I didn't know if anyone else in the family took this seriously, but I fully intended to adhere to her final wishes. Whether we buried or burned the old gal, somewhere in her future was a gold-plated epitaph engraved with those exact words.

In Edwardian Script font for a touch of class.

★★★

Mom was relaying a discussion she had with Nanna on Thanksgiving morning. This was how she preferred to speak with her mother— over the phone, thousands of blissful miles between them.

"I had to get off the phone with her, Jen. Your grandmother was on a rant. 'Why did Tom leave JoAnn?' she was screaming, 'I have a good mind to call him up and ask him.'"

"So I said, 'Yeah, and while we're at it, let's bring Daddy back from the dead and ask him why he was such a miserable son of a bitch for most of his life.'" Mom snorted. I heard dishes being washed in the background.

"Mom . . . " I chastised.

"Well, I'll never get the yams and green beans finished if I'm on the phone with her all day. She was in a mood."

"She's always in a mood. That's what I love about her. You should be recording every conversation you have with that woman. I, for one, take copious notes."

★★★

"What does this look like to you?"

What preceded this question was her painfully slow walk down the center aisle of the pharmacy I worked at just out of high school. The rather rotund woman gripped dual walking sticks, knocking items off the lower shelves on either side of her as she moved. Scarlett Kaufmann, we'll call her, so as not to be sued. She was a regular customer. Regular meaning often—she was by no means *regular*.

Pharmacy Technician was my title, but indentured servant to a mob of regular senior citizen customers was what should have been printed on my resume. Before I had children and my job description became Human Kleenex, I actually had gainful employment whereby I received a weekly paycheck.

Scarlett, like most of our customers, habitually availed herself of the knowledgeable pharmacists, who spent most of their time ducked down behind the counter to avoid such confrontations.

Pharmacists are not doctors. Sure, they can tell you anything you want to know about most medications listed in the Physicians Desk Reference, but they are decidedly not diagnosticians.

The customers, however, did not understand the distinction. To them, these men and women in white lab coats were a free source of information— usually the second stop after having called a few relatives and relayed their particular signs and symptoms over the phone. Having not come to a satisfactory determination via familial means, their next trip was to the local pharmacy.

By the time Scarlett made it halfway up the aisle, I'd doubled back behind her and began gathering the items left in her slow wake. She reminded me of a manatee— one of the large, friendly mammals common to the intercoastal Florida waterways.

I could see the pharmacist, a man who would later become my future *first* husband, wither under the harsh glare of the fluorescent store lights. She approached the wall separating the pharmacist from impending doom, grabbing the register for support, breathing heavily due to her long journey from her car to the rear of the store.

What she did next will be seared into my brain for all of eternity. I now believe it was moments like these that prepared me for the children I have today.

Unfortunately, I'd made it around the counter and was standing behind the wall next to the pharmacist, facing her as she lifted up the massive amounts of material she called a blouse. I froze as events seemed to play out in slow motion. She hung one of her walking sticks on the metal wiring of the impulse section, then grabbed the underwire of a bra I can only describe as colossal, and heaved it over both breasts, only managing to pin both plump piles down like smashed water balloons.

The effect was awe inspiring, if not equally grotesque. Her large, floppy breasts, now plastered, half in and half out of the wiring, left her midsection in full view of the entire pharmacy department.

As she worked at keeping the blouse and bra up, one breast escaped further, the mud-colored nipple dangerously protruding from under the bra. I assume, over her double chins and mound of material covered flesh, she was unable to see her physical faux-pas and didn't know we were all privy to half of her saucer-sized areola.

"What does this look like to you?" With her thumb, she motioned to the vast area under her barely caged breasts, at what looked like a nasty rash.

Or scabies, possibly some flesh-eating virus?

I had no idea *what* was going on there, but it wasn't pretty. Red pustules, scaly patches, and a few scabs thrown in for good measure.

I felt certain I'd be skipping lunch.

The pharmacist-slash-future husband, though certainly as horrified as I, didn't miss a beat.

"Looks like a trip to the dermatologist might be a good idea."

"Don'cha got some kind of cream I can put on it?" Scarlett hadn't pulled her shirt down yet, and I felt the bile rising up my esophagus, along with an impending fit of giggles.

As I squatted to the floor, grabbing his leg for support and burying my face in his pant leg, the pharmacist left her with the last piece of advice he'd offer her that day.

"Ms. Kaufmann, I'm not a doctor, but even I can see there's nothing on my shelves that'll take care of that. Make an appointment with your doctor or go over to the ER and let them take a look at it."

I almost bit his calf through his pant leg as I tried to keep from exploding. At the same time, my coworker entered from the back room and saw me practically gnawing on our boss's leg.

"What's going on?" Inga asked in her thick German accent.

I could only point upward, in the direction I knew Scarlett stood, on the other side of the pharmacy counter. I watched as Inga raised herself on her tiptoes and stared at the customer over the counter.

"Oh, Jesus!" she exclaimed.

The pharmacist shook his leg, trying to detach me, and I crawled past the drug hoppers, still unable to compose myself.

It was only a few seconds, but I knew Scarlett was beating her not so hasty retreat because I could hear boxes of medication and other items falling to the floor on the aisles as she passed, mumbling under her breath.

Scarlett, and many others, unknowingly prepared me for Jake and his series of unfortunate, if not amusing, questions I am forced to field daily.

"Mom, why do they put pockets in the back of jeans?" Jake was bent over in front of my full length mirror, checking out his rear end. It was seven-fifteen in the morning, and we were just about out the door on our way to school.

"Huh?" I filled my coffee cup in the nearby kitchen.

"Why do they put pockets back there? It's stupid. If you put anything in them, you have to touch your butt to get it out. That's gross."

"Men usually put their wallets in their back pockets."

Jake thought about this as he slid his hands slowly into his back pockets.

"Girls are lucky. They have purses. They don't have to touch their butts."

I supposed his reasoning was sound, but I sighed because I knew what was coming next.

"I can't have a purse, right?" He was looking at his hands, deep inside the pockets.

"Well, you could if you wanted one, but I'm not sure it's the best idea in the world."

I could just picture him heading down the school hallway, an Yves St. Lauren bag over one shoulder, his backpack over the other.

"Do I have to wash my hands after I touch my butt?" Jake pulled his hands out of his back pockets and stared at them.

"No, I think the jean material between your butt and hands is plenty of germ protection, Jake."

I checked the clock—five minutes until the daily loading of backpacks and unwilling children into the car commenced.

"Touch your butt, Mom."

What's this, now?

"Huh?"

"Touch your butt so I can see you don't wash your hands after."

He was deep within a cycle: show me, don't tell me. *Repeat what I need you to repeat before I am able to do anything else*, was what he was thinking.

I slapped my palms on both butt cheeks and rubbed up and down ferociously, then held out my hands for his perusal.

"Wanna smell?" I offered.

"Ugh, Mom. You're so gross."

He grabbed his backpack and headed for the mud room, looking over his shoulder at me as I led his brother toward the door.

"Mom, I think you should wash your hands." Meaning, *I think I should wash my hands.*

"No, I'm good, thanks."

"Are you sure?" His hand was on the doorknob. We were seconds from exiting, but he didn't look . . . certain.

"Yep, pretty sure."

"Touch your butt one more time, to be sure."

I reached around him, opening the door and gently but firmly shoved him onto the front porch. I was making headway, albeit painfully slow headway.

"Jake, you're killing me, here."

"Please! Do it!"

Jaxson was already running for the car, so I decided to humor him.

"Fine." I set my coffee cup on the ledge and slapped both palms on my sweatpant-clad ass cheeks for the second time that morning, rubbing hard enough to ignite a fire.

Then, I held my hands out for his inspection.

He stared at them for a couple of seconds.

"Are we good?" I asked, grabbing my coffee and taking a swig.

"Yeah, I guess."

Good.

December 14, 2009
Normal
By Jake Lopez

I think when people first see me not knowing me, I think they want to be mean to me. I don't like it. Not everyone but most of them. That's what I think. Sometimes when I see people doing stuff at school, I think that's what I should do. I do that all of the time. I feel like other kids can get away with it, which they do.

Kids at school make pig noises at only me. I hate it. I don't like my school. I feel nervous at school and I miss you a lot Mom and I didn't feel like I knew anyone and was going to be left forever at school when I was in kindergarten.

I have a very unlucky school life.

I just think that's what to do when I see other people acting mad, sad or any emotion. I don't understand why people hate me when I didn't do anything to them. And the people sometimes make me nervous because I don't know what to do. I wish I was at school with nobody but me so I would like school.

Now that I know I am autistic I don't want people to bother me. Before I didn't care because I thought I was a normal kid, but now I get more mad about it. If I never knew I was autistic I would have had a better life in middle school and no one would know I got mad in the past.

Also, I won't like to say this but I will. Sometimes skin grosses me out. People's bodies. Sometimes. I try to ignore it and it works sometimes. I think sometimes it's gross and I avoid it. And just to tell you, some things on faces too (pimples.) But it does not bother me anymore. Just sometimes when I look at Cody.

I wanted to tell you so don't even talk about it because it is not important Mom. When Ms. Chipman first saw me at the elementary school I thought real hard about how did she feel about me. When she was working with Jaxson's class. Now that I am in middle school, probably she sees me get mad and now she doesn't like me anymore.

The Weight of Normal

Autism isn't something a person has, or a "shell" that a person is trapped inside. There's no normal child hidden behind the autism. Autism is a way of being. It is pervasive—it colors every experience, every sensation, perception, thought, emotion, and encounter, every aspect of existence. It is not possible to separate the autism from the person—and if it were possible, the person you'd have left would not be the same person you started with.

—*from* Don't Mourn for Us, by Jim Sinclair

As a parent, I was lucky enough to understand, right from the outset, that grieving for what my children *weren't* wasn't productive. But many parents of autistic children go through a grieving process as they deal with their own shattered preconceptions.

I have very vivid memories of the day Jaxson was diagnosed. The appointment with the doctor was a doozy. Once out of the waiting room filled with toys, we were relegated to a small room and the door shut behind us. Jax does not like being in a confined space against his will. It was the middle of summer in Florida, and the pediatrician's little waiting room was oppressively hot. It only took minutes before Jaxson began ripping off his clothes and screaming, trying to get out the door.

As my mother and I waited for his doctor to come in and begin the assessment, Jaxson clawed at me, cried, and pulled my hair as I blocked his exit. Both of us were clammy, uncomfortable, and more than a bit frightened. I ended up with bleeding claw marks across my chest, only the beginning of my body as a battlefield—each nick and scar a landmark on the roadmap of our lives together.

Jax was causing such a ruckus that the pediatrician came in after hearing banging on the walls, "What's going on in here?"

"I'm sorry." I felt pitifully unequal to the task of managing my, then, four-year-old child. He was completely nonverbal, only able to communicate by pointing and grunting.

"It's fine," the pediatrician sat on a stool and watched Jaxson for a few minutes as I did my best not to break down and cry.

What followed was a questionnaire used as a diagnostic tool—a points system attributed to different developmental milestones. Some of these included motor skills, social interaction, eye contact, responsiveness to verbal cues, resistance to change in routine, abnormal ways of relating with others, and tantrums.

Jaxson passed with flying colors. He was, indeed, autistic.

There were to be future meetings where he would be observed for a period of time over the summer by a team specializing in developmental disabilities, but on that day, my suspicions were confirmed. I'd already done enough research and scoured enough books to know, in my heart, what I was dealing with.

At that point, even Jake, four years older than his brother, had not been diagnosed properly. We'd tried two other pediatricians and nobody had any answers for me, presumably because of Jake's high-functioning status. He'd slipped through the cracks, but I knew. It would take another year and a move out of state to get Jake a proper diagnosis to confirm what I already knew.

But on *that* day, Jaxson's diagnosis day, reality sunk in. Sometimes, reality bites.

I had two autistic children.

On the car ride home, I felt a sort of relief. But when I looked over at my Mom, she was crying.

"What's wrong?" I asked.

"Now we know. He's autistic." She swallowed hard.

"But Mom. Jax is the same kid we entered the doctor's office with this morning. Right?"

To her credit, Mom saw the truth of this viewpoint almost instantaneously. She's the best advocate for my children that I could ask for.

Not all parents and family members get to this point as quickly. After diagnosis, they are left to adjust to a relationship with a very different child than the one they fantasized about during the nine-month gestation period.

I understand this feeling.

But, maybe because of how I was raised, I was never disappointed that my children were different. I loved that Jax would smile when I rubbed my elbow on his cheek. As a toddler, he used it as a touchstone. He'd walk over, bend my arm for me, and put his hands around the crook of my arm, rubbing my elbow all around his face.

Later, his musical inclinations thrilled me.

"We, woo, we, woo wa-ki." Eight-year-old Jaxson came running out of his room, on a mission to retrieve a juice box, singing gibberish words to a tune I immediately recognized.

"We, woo, we, woo wa-ki," he continued as my head snapped around in disbelief.

We will, we will, rock you!

Queen. Are you kidding me?

I resolved to play the Beatles more frequently, because if Jax could parrot lines from *SpongeBob* and *Jimmy Neutron*, surely he could sing along to "Hey Jude" or "While My Guitar Gently Weeps."

Even his tantrums had the ability to make me smile.

One Thanksgiving, I'd pulled out the pink mixing bowl to begin preparing the stuffing and because he associated that particular bowl with my fantastic taco salad, he immediately presumed that's what I was making.

"Taco sa-wid?" he asked, and then looked into the bowl, only to find breadcrumbs, celery, walnuts, apples and onions.

He furrowed his brow.

"Nope. It's Thanksgiving, buddy. I'm making stuffing. Look, see the turkey?" I opened the oven.

Jax bent over and sniffed. "Oh, yuck!"

Okay, so that's a no on the turkey for you then?

"Yuck. No tuh-kee. Oh, yuck!" He slammed his foot on the floor and placed his fists on his hips—quite the insolent little stance. I blamed Cartoon Network.

He smacked my arm and threw himself on the floor, screaming.

"No hitting, Jaxson. That's not nice."

"No, not nice. No." He was repeating whatever I said as he kicked me in the shins. I closed the oven door to keep us both from getting third degree burns and a nice holiday visit to the emergency room.

When he kicked me a third time, I grabbed his ankle. "No, sir!"

"No, no, sir!" he yelled, adding a military salute.

I have no idea where he'd seen it done, but it was pretty funny.

"Heil Hitler!" I laughed, one arm outstretched. When he repeated it, I immediately regretted my flippancy. That wasn't something I wanted him repeating at school, or anywhere for that matter.

With Jake's miraculous imagination, I regularly marvel at the questions he asks or the things he says.

"I love that Chef Ravioli, Mom. It has magic meat because it's so tasty!"

Yes, indeedy!

Sure, there were, and still are, cringe-worthy moments.

One Halloween, Will and I took the boys to a pumpkin patch. Jake was five and Jax was only one. I carried the little guy, while my husband led Jake around, looking for the perfect gourd.

As I scanned the area, I heard the distinct sound of water trickling from somewhere. To my horror, I turned in time to see Jake, pants around his ankles, peeing right on a pumpkin.

My eyes darted back and forth as I hissed at Will, "Psst. Pick one and let's go."

There was a very brief but harried discussion as to whether we should tell someone about the now urine-covered pumpkin, purchase it ourselves, or just get the hell out of there.

I'm ashamed to say we chose the latter after paying for our own piss-free pumpkin.

The cringe-worthy moments weren't as bad as the black moments—moments when I wasn't sure I'd even make it through another day without having a mental breakdown. But, eventually, I developed a new normal, a way of not only existing, but understanding the benefits of seeing the beauty in the surreal.

It wasn't, and still isn't, as easy for their father. My mantra to him is always, "You have to love the children you have, not the ones you wish you had."

He went through that grieving process, eventually realizing neither of his kids would play Little League, or enjoy accompanying him to Yankees games. He plowed through the stages of grief as I played hall monitor.

Denial—"There's nothing wrong with them a little discipline won't cure."

I could actually hear Doctor Phil in my head, *"Yeah? So how's that workin' for ya'?"*

Anger—"What did I do?" or "What did *you* do?" or "Why me?"

Well, why *not* you? There is pain and suffering everywhere, so what about *you* is so special that you'd be any less inclined to have something challenging enter your life? It could always be worse.

Depression—He spent hours playing dominoes and drinking with his family, while I got a prescription for Lexapro.

Acceptance—This one's the most important—a step I've mastered and he's still working on.

There is a difference between resignation and acceptance. You have to eat what's on your plate, not shove it around until it resembles something else.

But, you've really made it when you can find the good that comes out of the pain. Pain and joy are equally necessary in life— without one, you wouldn't be able to recognize the other.

What I've learned about life is that it's about getting from point A to point B but everyone does this differently. The path of one person might take them past a goat sacrifice, while another might include a pit stop, hunched naked over a mirror, checking their lower orifice for poop residue.

Though each path is different, every journey unique, we all enter the world via the female uterus, and exit it once we stop breathing.

Everything between the two is up for grabs.

With each living person, history is left to judge what their contribution to the world might be. Labels, supposedly, inform who we are, but the beauty of life is that it enables us to accept or reject them at will. We can allow others to define us, or decide for ourselves who we really are.

It is of far greater consequence when we step outside the box than when we remain where others think we belong— a nice, tidy package wrapped in familiar paper.

By all means, stay in your box if that's where you feel most comfortable, but don't concern yourself if someone else jumps out of theirs, bends over and takes a crap on it, douses it with lighter fluid, and watches it illuminate the sky.

To each, his own.

Autistic persons are often defined by their failure to use language and perceive their surroundings in the expected way.

Expected is the operative word here.

It is presumed that there has been some disturbance in their psychological development so their reaction to stimuli, their personal interpretations of the world, and formations of relationships follow unusual patterns.

Unusual is the operative word here.

I welcome the unexpected— thrive on the unusual. If only *these* were the definition of normal—unexpected, unusual—then the use of labels would cease to exist.

That is a day I look forward to with relish . . .

. . . atop a banana, with a bit of mayo, cilantro, peanut butter, and liver paté.

But that's not normal, you say?

Well, I say, Normal's just a town in Illinois, south of Peoria, and north of Bloomington.

A friend recently told me I was lucky to have my life, "While you're enjoying an eight-course meal, most people are sitting down with a frozen dinner."

Profundity: you can't find it in the frozen food section.

Acknowledgements

*A*hem . . .

I'd like to thank the Academy . . . oh, wait—that's the wrong speech. Let me dig around in my purse next to the three-year-old cough drop covered in fuzz and the crumpled emergency band-aid, to retrieve my scrawled notes with regard to anyone who has ever helped me, moved me, inspired me, laughed with (or at) me—basically anyone who has rubbed up against me along the way.

You should probably get comfy because I'm not working against a thirty-second time constraint so this could take awhile. Pretend I'm Dame Judy Densch—no award show music conductor would dare to shoo her off the stage with annoying theme music, and this dame expects the same treatment.

Under the category of inspirational people, I must start with my aunt, Mary Decker Osborne. She is responsible for sparking an interest in me that has, time and again, kept me from taking a disposable razor to my wrists.

Okay, don't oversell it, drama queen.

Some sort of peculiar alchemy took hold as I clutched the unbound pages of one of her early manuscripts because at eleven years old I instantly knew:

This is what I want to be.

That stack of paper containing thousands of words she'd banged out on her Smith Corona whispered in my ear—a secret I've been trying to decipher ever since—though to this day I cannot remember a single sentence of the book. I only remember marveling at the weight of that unbound manuscript and knowing something about myself I hadn't known moments earlier.

For years I watched manuscript pages pile up on my own desk (and in my hard drive) along with their accompanying rejection letters. Then one day I popped out a kid and I was suddenly doing less writing and more diaper changing. Another kid came four years later—long enough later for me to realize something strange was going on in my household.

When Jake's pediatrician failed to give me the answers I needed, I began researching his symptoms. My firstborn was quirky from day one, but eventually I figured out that his quirkiness probably had a diagnosis attached:

Autism.

Once Jaxson was born, my writing took a further back seat to mining for poo pebbles hidden in every corner of my house, dealing with aggressive behavioral outbursts, OCD, and a shit-storm of other symptoms that left me laughing uproariously when I wasn't curled in the fetal position on the bathroom floor, sobbing. I continued to write whenever I could, my ass glued to the computer chair for fifteen minute intervals, between unnatural disasters like septic system overflows and wayward autistic children finding their way onto the roof of my house.

It wasn't until my boys were twelve and eight years old that someone said to me, "You should write about your life. It's kind of funny. When it's not depressing as hell."

So I did, one story at a time, sharing each chapter hot off the press with other writers on my workshop site, The Next Big Writer. (Thanks, Sol!)

I owe a huge debt of gratitude to those early readers who suggested changes, helped with editing, and most importantly, shared their own stories of familial dysfunction. I'd like to thank Paul Negri (who went above and beyond, so to him I owe a debt I probably will never be able to repay), Mitch Geller (who pushed me to swim deeper when it was clear I was treading water with regard to certain topics), Kat Nove, (whom I've cowritten a book with and can tell you with certainty is funnier than I could ever hope to be). She is also my closest friend and the one person I rant to daily via email. Pattie Ann Yeager (who has an autistic child in her family and shared Lego horror stories), and Michael Amrein (an amazing cop and father who traded funny and gut-wrenching stories with me, and has since passed). He said to me more than once, "Jen, you ain't right." I will always remember him as someone who made me smile and will miss him very much.

The list of writing comrades goes on—a committed group who helped make this book better with each draft: Rachel Hamm, Michelle Montgomery, John Hamler, Sara Basrai, Ama Adjapon, Jeanne Bannon, Tirzah L. Goodwin, Scott Eberhart, Nathan Childs, Ann Elle Altman, Sabrina Dalton, Doug Moore, Dennis Hart, Molly Winter, Amy Metz, Louise Saville, Wendy Squire, Jane Jones, Sue Hall, Dwight Okita, and my mom . . .

Speaking of Mommy Dearest (who is like my kids and my hemorrhoids—both occasionally a pain in the ass)—her brand of rabid maternal support has served me well over the years. She's also a fantastic grandmother. She and my stepfather, Bob, helped us move from Florida to Michigan when my kids weren't getting the educational opportunities they deserved, and their lives have greatly improved because of it.

Which brings us to teachers, paraprofessionals and other school support staff. The village it takes to raise my children is as vast and far reaching as most right wing conspiracies (and talking points). I'm not sure if some teachers realize they can make or break a child for life with a well chosen (or badly chosen) word or deed. Teachers and hairdressers are the two people you don't want to be sitting in front of if they have an inherent distaste for their chosen occupation. While the latter will probably just cost you a month or so of bad hair days, the former can do far more damage—for a far longer period of time. Like forever.

I get that teachers don't get paid enough. In fact, in my utopia, teacher pay raises would be subsidized by the immediate rerouting of one-third of all income made by professional basketball, baseball, and football players. (Yeah, yeah—address your hate mail to God. I haven't got the time or inclination to argue about it. It's my utopian ideal and I'm sticking to it.) Having said that, if you're a teacher and don't like what you do, do everyone a favor and find another career. The job is too important to be squandered by someone who's just doing time.

Luckily, in the teacher category, my kids have mostly drawn the longer straws. Their lives have benefited tremendously from the caring individuals we've had the privilege to work with over the years. It began with Miss Markley, Jake's kindergarten teacher. One day she handed me a newspaper article which speculated that Einstein had been on the autism spectrum.

"This might be something to look into," she said.

Wait, the genius thing or the autistic thing?

I got the answer from her concerned facial expression. I have to say, if you're going to hear that kind of news about your child (at three in the afternoon when you still have four loads of dirty laundry waiting for you at home), having your child compared to Einstein is a lot better than, say, Hitler. So thanks to her for the time, patience, and soft-serve diagnosis. That was the day I started my Internet research on autism.

Jake did not reap the benefits of Early Intervention like Jaxson did. When we reached Michigan, my little guy was gently subjected to an evaluation by a team of experts, and then enrolled in a three-hour-a-day preschool program for children with developmental delays. Michelle Welch, Becky Luce, and Mrs. Beckwith ushered Jaxson through his first school experience. They were loving, qualified, knowledgeable and firm—all qualities needed to adequately deal with children on the autism spectrum. Here we also met speech therapist Kathy Connor, occupational therapist Marty Guiney, social worker Cindy Warner, psychologist Deborah Mako, and supervisor Pat Langworthy, who all continue to work with my boys on their education goals.

Their ASD teachers nurture as they educate, helping my boys bloom and grow into fine little men. Huge thanks to Cindy Swymeler and Cindy DesJardins, as well as their support staff, Linda Chipman, Kathy Tilmann, Donna Scott, Ginny Waite, Mrs. Dyer and Mr. Draper, Jan Cassidy and Dan Weshe.

Many thanks to Dawn the fabulous van driver who escorted my kids safely to and from school for a time.

There are a great many General Education teachers who have taken the time to get to know my children. In Jake's case, for instance, the middle school gym teacher who still shoots baskets one-on-one with Jake when he's feeling stressed, and the computer teacher who spent the first ten minutes of middle school orientation discussing his handlebar moustache with Jake—because my child simply couldn't move on through his orientation until he found out how his future computer teacher got his facial hair to curl up so magnificently. Now Jake knows everything anyone needs to know about moustache wax. I'm not sure how much he knows about computers—other than how to look up video game cheat codes—but if the topic of facial hair ever comes up, Jake will be able to effectively navigate the conversation.

Jake has forbidden me from naming specific general education teachers and I will respect that. (At thirteen, he doesn't want any of his current teachers thinking he actually has an affinity for them. God forbid.)

At the elementary school level, I'd like to thank general education teachers Heidi Mellema, Tracy Hansen, Mrs. Boltze, Robbie Siegel, Mrs. McDonald and Mr. Emington (gym), Mrs. Krantz (art) and Mr. David the music teacher. I am grateful to the entire staff of G.T Norman Elementary and Reed City Middle School for their support.

A huge *muchas gracias* goes to my husband Will—the breadwinner, sperm donor and all-around nice guy who, even though he thinks the best time to get rowdy with the children is two seconds before bedtime, has worked hard at deciphering his kids wants and needs and always does his best to provide for them. He's a good guy and I don't tell him that often enough.

We both owe my editor, Jennifer McCartney, a special thank you. She has a deft editing hand and a good sense of how humor needs to play out on the page. Most importantly, during the editing process, her questions about clarifying our relationship for the reader led to a discussion between Will and I that was long overdue. We now know where we stand—even though neither of us are living in what we'd consider the ideal Shangri-la, it's *our* Shangri-la and we're "in it to win it" as far as our kids are concerned.

A lifetime of thanks goes to my sister Resi, who gets me better than anyone else in the world. That's something you're lucky if you get in life—one person who knows you to your core and still loves you.

I would be remiss if I didn't thank my Nanna, Concetta Angelina Morizzio Stec, for assuring me, as far back as I can remember, that I was going to be a famous writer one day. Even though I knew it wasn't true, it's always nice to hear, even if you're hearing it from someone whose favorite shows are *Judge Judy* and *Walker, Texas Ranger,* and swears to the factual validity of every story she reads in the *National Enquirer.* Nanna's a loudmouthed Italian woman rapidly bearing down on ninety and I credit her DNA as being a major ingredient in the recipe that is me. The woman is a delicious little malapropism wrapped in a Depends undergarment and she's one of my favorite people in the world.

Take that, Oprah. "My Favorite Things" list includes my Nanna, Preparation-H, chocolate, McDonald's Iced Mochas, and Rachel Maddow (not necessarily in that order), all of which regularly delivers the yum factor to one of my orifices, or my teetering sanity.

Finally, I want to thank my children for changing me from the person I was to the person I was meant to be. I started this journey we call life as an introverted little shadow and now I'm a very loud, often obnoxious voice—perfectly remade to advocate for my children, and anyone else who hasn't quite found their voice . . . yet.

Cue the cheesy music . . .